Psoriasis - Pathogenesis, Clinical Features, and Treatment

Edited by Selda Pelin Kartal

Published in London, United Kingdom

Psoriasis - Pathogenesis, Clinical Features, and Treatment
http://dx.doi.org/10.5772/intechopen.1008602
Edited by Selda Pelin Kartal

Contributors
Ammar Al-Dujaili, Arnulfo-Hernán Nava-Zavala, Aylin Türel Ermertcan, Belal Muwafak, Columba-Julieta Navarro-Romero, Daniel O. Costache, Georgina Vega-Fregoso, Hayder Al-Darraji, Maria Magdalena Constantin, Mihaela Georgescu, Muhammed Ali Mergen, Mustafa Ekici, Mădălina Mariana Motoacă, Rasha Aoun, Sandra Guzmán-Silahua, Selda Pelin Kartal, Shaimaa Farouk, Tubanur Çetinarslan, Tuğcan Yüksek

First published in London, United Kingdom, 2025 by IntechOpen
IntechOpen is the global imprint of INTECHOPEN LIMITED, registered in England and Wales, registration number: 11086078, 167-169 Great Portland Street, London, W1W 5PF, United Kingdom

For EU product safety concerns: IN TECH d.o.o., Prolaz Marije Krucifikse Kozulić 3, 51000 Rijeka, Croatia, info@intechopen.com or visit our website at intechopen.com.

British Library Cataloguing-in-Publication Data
A catalogue record for this book is available from the British Library

Psoriasis - Pathogenesis, Clinical Features, and Treatment
Edited by Selda Pelin Kartal
p. cm.
Print ISBN 978-1-83635-121-4
Online ISBN 978-1-83635-120-7
eBook (PDF) ISBN 978-1-83635-122-1

If disposing of this product, please recycle the paper responsibly.

Meet the editor

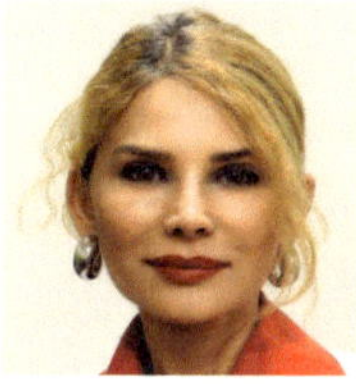

Selda Pelin Kartal graduated from Hacettepe University School of Medicine. Currently, she is a Professor and the Head of the Department of Dermatology at the University of Health Sciences, Ministry of Health, Etlik City Hospital in Ankara, Turkey. She has co-authored over 200 published articles and supervised several master's and postdoctoral students. Her actual interests are focused on acne, psoriasis, urticaria, autoimmune bullous diseases, Behçet's disease and cosmetic dermatology.

Contents

Preface

This book aims to provide readers with a comprehensive overview of psoriasis, including its pathogenesis, clinical features, and treatment options. It is created by experts in various fields, who aim to expand knowledge about psoriasis. I am grateful to all the contributors and leading experts for submitting their excellent work, which provides an in-depth view of all aspects of the content, backed by the most current literature in the field. I would like to extend special thanks to Publishing Process Manager Laura Divić for bringing the book to its current form, and to my sons, Demir Durmazlar and Ares, for their understanding and patience during the time I spent away from them.

Dr. Selda Pelin Kartal
Professor,
Department of Dermatology and Venereology,
University of Health Science,
Ministry of Health Etlik City Hospital,
Ankara, Turkey

Chapter 1

Lifestyle and Nutrition in Psoriasis: Key Factors in Pathogenesis and Disease Modulation

Shaimaa Farouk, Rasha Aoun, Belal Muwafak, Hayder Al-Darraji and Ammar Al-Dujaili

Abstract

Psoriasis is a chronic, immune-mediated inflammatory skin disease with systemic implications and complex multifactorial pathogenesis. While genetic and immunologic mechanisms are central to disease development, increasing attention has been given to the role of lifestyle and nutrition in modulating disease onset, severity, and response to therapy. This chapter provides a comprehensive overview of the current evidence linking modifiable lifestyle factors—diet, obesity, smoking, alcohol use, stress, and physical activity—to psoriasis pathophysiology. Particular attention is given to the impact of Western dietary patterns, pro-inflammatory adipokines, and the gut-skin axis in mediating systemic inflammation. The chapter highlights key nutritional components, such as omega-3 fatty acids, antioxidants, and dietary fiber, which may play protective roles, and explores the detrimental effects of alcohol and smoking on disease progression and therapeutic efficacy. Pediatric, pregnant, lactating and geriatric psoriasis is discussed in the context of early dietary exposures, obesity, and psychosocial stressors. Recent clinical trials assessing lifestyle interventions—including dietary modification, weight reduction, and stress management—are critically reviewed. Through an integrative lens, this chapter emphasizes the importance of incorporating lifestyle-based strategies into the management of psoriasis. For dermatologists, this evidence underscores the value of addressing modifiable risk factors alongside pharmacologic treatment to improve outcomes, enhance quality of life, and reduce the long-term burden of comorbidities.

Keywords: psoriasis, lifestyle, nutrition, pathogenesis, obesity

1. Introduction

Psoriasis is a common, chronic inflammatory dermatosis affecting 2–3% of the global population and is associated with significant systemic, metabolic, and psychological comorbidities [1, 2]. Traditionally regarded as a dermatological condition driven by immune dysregulation and genetic predisposition, psoriasis is now understood to be a systemic disease characterized by chronic inflammation involving the interleukin (IL)-23/IL-17 axis, T-helper (Th) cells, and a wide network of cytokines [3].

IntechOpen

In parallel with advances in immunobiology, there has been growing recognition of the substantial impact of modifiable lifestyle factors on disease expression and outcomes. Dietary habits, body weight, smoking, alcohol use, stress, and physical activity all contribute to systemic inflammation and immune activity—core mechanisms in psoriasis pathogenesis [4–6]. Importantly, many of these factors are prevalent in psoriatic populations and are increasingly viewed not only as comorbidities but also as contributors to disease severity and poor therapeutic response [7, 8].

Nutrition, in particular, has emerged as a crucial yet often overlooked component in psoriasis care. Western dietary patterns, characterized by high intake of saturated fats, simple carbohydrates, and processed foods, have been linked to increased inflammatory markers and psoriasis flares. In contrast, anti-inflammatory diets rich in fruits, vegetables, whole grains, and polyunsaturated fatty acids may help reduce disease activity [9, 10]. Additionally, obesity and metabolic syndrome—frequent in psoriatic patients—further amplify inflammation through adipokine and insulin-mediated pathways (**Figure 1**) [11].

This diagram summarizes how obesity, smoking, psychological stress, alcohol use, and a Western diet contribute to chronic psoriasis by promoting systemic inflammation through mechanisms such as cytokine activation, oxidative stress, gut permeability, and hormonal dysregulation.

This chapter aims to synthesize the latest evidence on how lifestyle and nutrition modulate psoriasis, integrating clinical, immunological, and metabolic perspectives. A particular focus is placed on the pediatric population and recent interventional trials. For specialist dermatologists, understanding the pathophysiological relevance of these factors is essential for delivering comprehensive, patient-centered care.

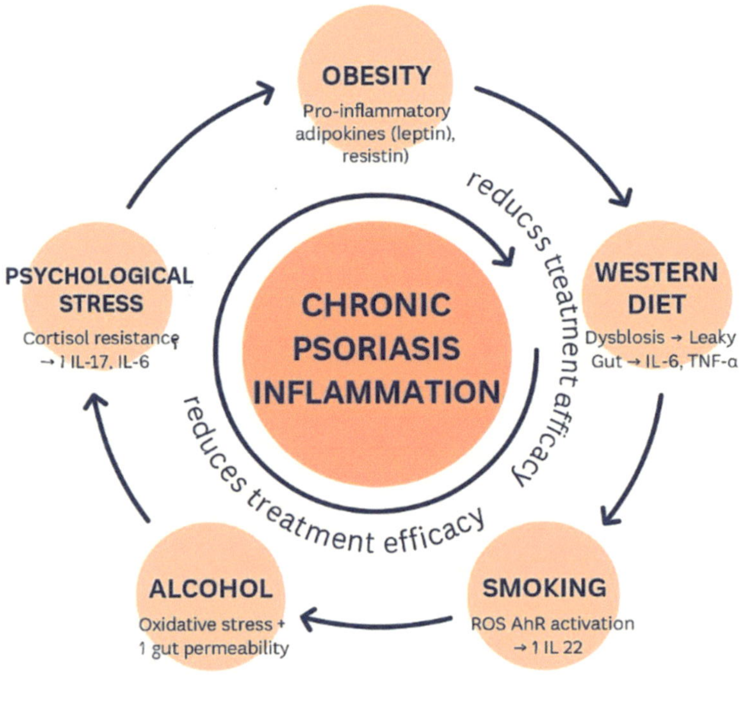

Figure 1.
Lifestyle factors driving chronic psoriasis inflammation.

2. The pathophysiological basis of psoriasis

Psoriasis is primarily driven by dysregulated innate and adaptive immune responses involving key inflammatory cytokines and cellular pathways. Central to its pathogenesis is the activation of dendritic cells, which stimulate Th1 and Th17 cell responses, leading to increased production of pro-inflammatory mediators such as tumor necrosis factor-alpha (TNF-α), IL-17, IL-22, and IL-23 [1–3]. These cytokines induce keratinocyte proliferation, angiogenesis, and recruitment of neutrophils, resulting in the characteristic psoriatic plaques.

Beyond cutaneous involvement, psoriasis is associated with systemic inflammation. Elevated levels of C-reactive protein (CRP), TNF-α, and IL-6 are frequently observed in psoriatic patients, indicating a state of chronic low-grade inflammation that contributes to cardiovascular disease, insulin resistance, and metabolic syndrome

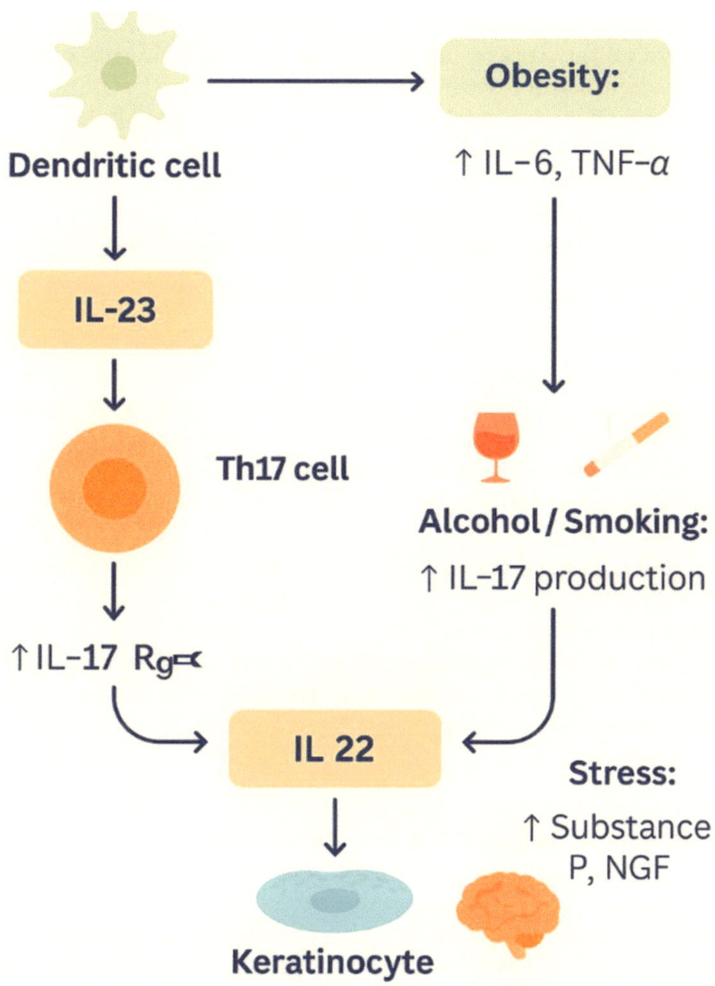

Figure 2.
IL-23/IL-17 pathway in psoriasis with lifestyle influence.

[4, 5]. The interaction between genetic predisposition and environmental triggers—including infection, stress, medications, and trauma (Koebner phenomenon)—initiates and perpetuates these immune responses.

Recent studies also highlight the role of the gut-skin axis and gut microbiota dysbiosis in psoriasis. Alterations in microbial composition may contribute to intestinal permeability and systemic immune activation, further linking lifestyle and dietary factors to disease activity [6, 7]. These insights underscore the importance of examining external influences—particularly lifestyle behaviors—as contributors to systemic immune dysregulation in psoriasis (**Figure 2**).

3. Obesity and metabolic dysregulation

Obesity is a significant and modifiable risk factor for both the development and progression of psoriasis. Numerous epidemiological studies demonstrate a positive association between body mass index (BMI) and psoriasis severity [8, 9]. Adipose tissue is not merely a fat-storage depot but an active endocrine organ that secretes adipokines (e.g., leptin and resistin) and pro-inflammatory cytokines, such as TNF-α, IL-6, and IL-1β, which can exacerbate psoriatic inflammation [10, 11].

Obese individuals exhibit increased levels of oxidative stress and systemic inflammation, both of which enhance immune dysregulation. In particular, leptin, which is elevated in obesity, promotes Th1 and Th17 differentiation and reduces regulatory T cell (Treg) activity, thereby sustaining chronic inflammation [12]. In contrast, adiponectin, which possesses anti-inflammatory properties, is typically reduced in obese psoriatic patients [13].

The association between psoriasis and metabolic syndrome—including dyslipidemia, hypertension, insulin resistance, and type 2 diabetes—is well-established. These conditions not only share common inflammatory pathways but also contribute to the high cardiovascular risk observed in psoriatic patients [14].

Importantly, lifestyle interventions aimed at reducing body weight have shown clinical benefit. Weight loss through caloric restriction, physical activity, or bariatric surgery is associated with significant reductions in Psoriasis Area and Severity Index (PASI) scores and improved response to biologic therapies [15, 16]. These findings highlight the relevance of addressing obesity as a central component in the holistic management of psoriasis (**Figure 2**).

IL-23 activates Th17 cells to produce IL-17A/F and IL-22, driving keratinocyte activation in psoriasis. Obesity, alcohol, and stress enhance this pathway, worsening inflammation through cytokine upregulation and mast cell activation.

4. Dietary influence on psoriasis pathogenesis

Diet is a powerful modulator of systemic inflammation and immune function, both of which are central to the pathogenesis of psoriasis. Epidemiological and interventional studies have demonstrated that dietary composition can significantly influence disease activity and therapeutic outcomes [1–3]. Western dietary patterns—marked by high intake of red and processed meats, saturated fats, simple carbohydrates, and ultra-processed foods—have been associated with increased psoriasis prevalence and severity [4].

DOI: http://dx.doi.org/10.5772/intechopen.1011490

These pro-inflammatory diets contribute to gut microbiota dysbiosis, promote oxidative stress, and increase the production of advanced glycation end-products (AGEs), all of which enhance systemic inflammation. High-glycemic diets, in particular, may exacerbate insulin resistance and promote a Th1/Th17 immune profile, further sustaining psoriatic inflammation [5, 6].

In contrast, anti-inflammatory diets—such as the Mediterranean diet—rich in vegetables, fruits, legumes, whole grains, fish, and extra virgin olive oil, have been associated with lower psoriasis activity and improved quality of life [7, 8]. These diets are high in polyphenols, fiber, and omega-3 fatty acids, all of which have immunomodulatory effects. Observational studies have found that higher adherence to the Mediterranean diet correlates with lower PASI scores and reduced systemic inflammation markers in psoriatic patients [9].

These findings suggest that dietary interventions may serve as a non-pharmacologic, adjunctive strategy to modulate disease severity and improve therapeutic response, particularly in patients with comorbid metabolic dysfunction.

4.1 Key dietary components and mechanisms

Several specific dietary components have been investigated for their potential roles in modulating psoriatic inflammation:

4.1.1 Omega-3 and omega-6 fatty acids

Omega-3 polyunsaturated fatty acids (PUFAs), found in fatty fish, flaxseed, and walnuts, have demonstrated anti-inflammatory properties through inhibition of arachidonic acid metabolism and suppression of IL-1, IL-6, and TNF-α production [10, 11]. Randomized controlled trials have reported improvements in erythema, scaling, and PASI scores in patients supplemented with fish oil [12].

In contrast, omega-6 PUFAs, prevalent in vegetable oils and processed foods, tend to promote pro-inflammatory eicosanoid synthesis. The balance between dietary omega-6 and omega-3 intake may therefore influence psoriatic activity [13].

4.1.2 Antioxidants and polyphenols

Oxidative stress is a key contributor to keratinocyte hyperproliferation and immune activation in psoriasis. Antioxidant-rich foods—such as berries, green tea, dark leafy vegetables, and extra virgin olive oil—help neutralize reactive oxygen species (ROS) and reduce inflammation [14, 15]. Polyphenols such as resveratrol and curcumin have been shown to downregulate NF-κB and STAT3 signaling pathways, which are central to psoriatic plaque development [16].

4.1.3 Vitamin D

Vitamin D plays an immunoregulatory role by enhancing Treg cell function and inhibiting Th17 responses. Psoriatic patients often have low serum levels of 25(OH)D, and supplementation has been associated with modest improvements in disease severity [17].

4.1.4 Gluten and celiac disease

An increased prevalence of celiac disease and gluten sensitivity has been reported among patients with psoriasis. Some studies suggest that gluten-free

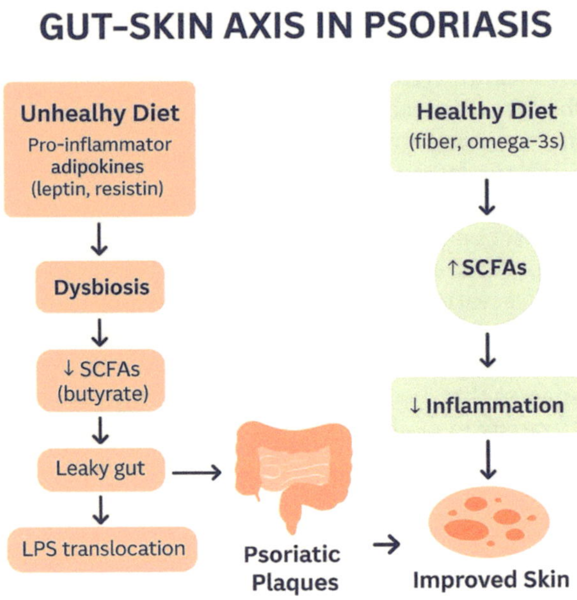

Figure 3.
Gut-skin axis disruption in psoriasis pathogenesis.

diets may improve psoriatic lesions in patients with anti-gliadin antibodies, though the evidence remains inconclusive [18, 19].

4.1.5 Fiber and the gut microbiota

Dietary fiber promotes a healthy gut microbiome and increases the production of short-chain fatty acids (SCFAs), which have anti-inflammatory effects and maintain intestinal barrier function. These mechanisms may indirectly influence systemic immune responses in psoriasis [20].

Together, these findings provide a compelling argument for targeted dietary interventions in psoriasis management, tailored to individual metabolic profiles and comorbid conditions (**Figure 3**).

An unhealthy diet leads to gut dysbiosis, reduced SCFAs, and leaky gut, triggering TLR4 activation and increased IL-6 and TNF-α. This promotes systemic inflammation and psoriatic plaques, which impair Treg function and perpetuate inflammation.

5. The role of alcohol and smoking

Alcohol and *smoking* are well-established environmental risk factors that influence the onset and progression of psoriasis. Both contribute to systemic inflammation, immune dysregulation, and impaired skin barrier function, ultimately exacerbating disease severity and undermining treatment outcomes.

Alcohol consumption has been associated with higher PASI scores, increased frequency of flares, and reduced responsiveness to systemic therapies [1, 2]. Ethanol promotes oxidative stress and impairs the gut barrier, allowing translocation of microbial products that activate immune cells and enhance systemic inflammation. Furthermore, alcohol induces keratinocyte proliferation and disrupts the skin's antimicrobial defense mechanisms [3]. Chronic consumption is particularly concerning in patients on hepatotoxic medications such as methotrexate, compounding liver toxicity risk [4].

Smoking is independently associated with increased psoriasis incidence and is particularly linked to pustular and palmoplantar variants [5]. Tobacco smoke promotes oxidative stress, increases levels of IL-1, IL-6, and TNF-α, and enhances neutrophilic activity—all contributing to psoriatic inflammation [6]. Nicotine itself can stimulate keratinocyte proliferation and angiogenesis *via* acetylcholine receptors on skin cells [7]. Importantly, smoking is a negative predictor of response to systemic and biologic treatments, particularly TNF-α inhibitors [8].

Clinically, both smoking cessation and alcohol reduction are essential lifestyle interventions that can improve psoriasis control, mitigate comorbid risks, and enhance treatment efficacy. These behaviors should be routinely addressed in dermatologic care, supported by motivational interviewing and multidisciplinary collaboration.

6. Psychological stress and neuroimmune modulation

Psychological stress is a recognized trigger and exacerbating factor in psoriasis, capable of inducing flares and contributing to chronic disease persistence. Stress activates the hypothalamic-pituitary-adrenal (HPA) axis, leading to increased levels of cortisol and catecholamines. While acutely adaptive, chronic stress results in immune dysregulation and altered cytokine profiles that promote inflammation [9, 10].

Neuroimmunological studies have demonstrated that stress enhances the production of neuropeptides (e.g., substance P and nerve growth factor), which activate mast cells, dendritic cells, and keratinocytes—further fueling psoriatic inflammation [11]. Additionally, chronic stress downregulates Treg cell function and skews T-cell responses toward Th1 and Th17 pathways, worsening immune-mediated disease [12].

The psychosocial burden of psoriasis itself—including stigmatization, depression, anxiety, and social withdrawal—can perpetuate a self-reinforcing cycle of stress and disease exacerbation. Psoriatic patients are at higher risk of mood disorders, and depression has been shown to correlate with increased CRP and TNF-α levels, reinforcing the bidirectional link between mental health and inflammation [13].

Stress-reduction interventions—including cognitive behavioral therapy (CBT), mindfulness-based stress reduction (MBSR), yoga, and relaxation techniques—have shown promise in improving quality of life and reducing flare frequency in psoriasis [14–16]. Integrating mental health support into dermatologic care is essential, particularly for patients with severe, recalcitrant, or early-onset disease.

7. Physical activity and immune regulation

Regular physical activity is a cornerstone of systemic health and plays a crucial role in modulating immune function and inflammation—two key elements in the pathogenesis and progression of psoriasis. Sedentary behavior is common among psoriatic patients, often due to discomfort, low self-esteem, or physical limitations caused by joint involvement or skin lesions [1]. However, the benefits of structured exercise extend well beyond physical conditioning and encompass metabolic, psychological, and immunological domains.

Physical activity has been shown to reduce circulating levels of pro-inflammatory cytokines, including TNF-α and IL-6, while increasing anti-inflammatory mediators such as IL-10 [2, 3]. Additionally, regular aerobic and resistance training improve insulin sensitivity, lower body mass index (BMI), and enhance endothelial function, all of which are relevant to the inflammatory and cardiovascular burden seen in psoriatic patients [4, 5].

Importantly, exercise also modulates stress reactivity by attenuating HPA axis hyperactivity and enhancing mood through increased release of endorphins and neurotransmitters like serotonin and dopamine [6]. These neuropsychological benefits are particularly valuable in a disease that often imposes significant emotional and social strain.

Nevertheless, dermatologists should counsel patients on appropriate exercise strategies, as excessive sweating, friction, and skin irritation may trigger Koebner's phenomenon in some individuals. Recommendations should include wearing breathable fabrics, maintaining skin hydration, and avoiding mechanical irritation. When integrated into a holistic care plan, physical activity can serve as a safe, accessible, and effective adjunctive therapy for psoriasis.

8. Pediatric psoriasis: Lifestyle factors and nutritional considerations

Pediatric psoriasis, affecting approximately 0.5–1% of children, presents unique challenges due to its early impact on physical, psychological, and social development. Like adult psoriasis, pediatric forms are influenced by both genetic and environmental factors, with emerging evidence pointing to a critical role for lifestyle and nutrition in disease expression and progression [7, 8].

Obesity is a particularly strong risk factor in children with psoriasis. Cross-sectional studies have shown that pediatric psoriasis is more prevalent in overweight and obese populations, with obesity often preceding disease onset [9]. Adiposity in childhood contributes to systemic inflammation through similar mechanisms observed in adults, including increased leptin and reduced adiponectin levels, which may enhance IL-17-mediated pathways [10].

Dietary quality in pediatric patients often mirrors that of the household, with Western-style diets rich in processed foods and sugars contributing to metabolic dysfunction. Nutritional interventions focusing on whole foods, fruits, vegetables, and omega-3 sources may offer immunological benefits and help maintain a healthy BMI [11, 12]. Early dietary counseling, involving both the child and caregivers, is critical for long-term disease management.

In addition, children with psoriasis may experience bullying, social withdrawal, and anxiety—all of which can exacerbate disease through psychoneuroimmune mechanisms. Addressing psychological stress in the pediatric population requires a sensitive, developmentally appropriate approach and may involve collaboration with pediatric psychologists or school counselors [13].

Given the lifelong implications of early-onset psoriasis, targeted lifestyle interventions in childhood may offer not only symptomatic relief but also long-term prevention of comorbidities such as metabolic syndrome, cardiovascular disease, and depression.

DOI: http://dx.doi.org/10.5772/intechopen.1011490

9. Psoriasis, lifestyle, and nutrition in pregnancy

Pregnancy represents a unique immunological state with significant shifts in inflammatory and hormonal pathways that can influence psoriasis activity. The maternal immune system undergoes a complex adaptation, favoring a Th2-dominant profile during gestation to support fetal tolerance, which often results in clinical improvement in Th1/Th17-mediated diseases such as psoriasis. However, the response is variable: while approximately 50% of women experience improvement, 25% report worsening of disease, and others remain stable [14].

Lifestyle and nutritional factors play a critical role in modulating psoriatic disease during pregnancy. Excessive maternal weight gain, poor glycemic control, and suboptimal nutritional intake may exacerbate systemic inflammation and negatively influence maternal and fetal outcomes. Additionally, gestational weight gain outside recommended ranges is associated with higher risks of hypertension, gestational diabetes, and adverse neonatal outcomes—all of which are more common in women with psoriasis [15].

Nutritional adequacy is especially important in psoriatic pregnancies. Deficiencies in folate, vitamin D, and omega-3 fatty acids—nutrients often found suboptimal in psoriasis patients—may impact both maternal disease and fetal development. Omega-3 fatty acids have anti-inflammatory properties and are essential for fetal neurodevelopment; adequate intake during pregnancy may confer benefits for maternal skin inflammation as well [16, 17].

Obesity is a particular concern. Women with psoriasis are more likely to enter pregnancy overweight or obese, and maternal adiposity increases the risk of disease flares, preeclampsia, and cesarean delivery [18]. Preconception counseling to optimize body weight and metabolic health is crucial for this patient population.

Smoking and alcohol use during pregnancy not only pose direct teratogenic risks but are also associated with greater disease severity and poorer maternal mental health. Dermatologists should work closely with obstetricians to counsel patients on the importance of lifestyle modifications before and during pregnancy.

Psychological stress is heightened during pregnancy and postpartum, and it may trigger or worsen psoriasis flares. Stress-reduction techniques such as prenatal yoga, mindfulness, and structured psychosocial support are safe, non-pharmacologic options that may benefit both maternal mental health and disease control.

Finally, *treatment decisions during pregnancy* must balance maternal disease severity with fetal safety. While lifestyle interventions are generally safe and encouraged, systemic therapies require careful selection. Lifestyle optimization can reduce the need for high-risk medications and may enhance the effectiveness of pregnancy-safe therapies.

Key clinical recommendations include:

- Preconception assessment of BMI, nutritional status, and lifestyle habits
- Counseling on anti-inflammatory diets and adequate intake of folate, vitamin D, and omega-3 s
- Smoking and alcohol cessation strategies
- Coordination with obstetric teams for integrated care
- Consideration of postpartum flare risks and mental health monitoring

10. Psoriasis and lactation: Implications of lifestyle and nutrition

Lactation represents a distinct physiological phase with unique implications for psoriasis management, nutritional requirements, and maternal well-being. Although relatively underexplored, emerging evidence suggests that the postpartum period may be associated with fluctuating disease activity, often influenced by hormonal changes, stress, and sleep disruption. While many women experience remission during pregnancy, the postpartum period is commonly associated with disease flare, potentially due to a rapid rebound in pro-inflammatory Th1/Th17 cytokine activity as estrogen and progesterone levels decline [19]. For lactating women with moderate to severe psoriasis, this can pose challenges for both maternal functioning and infant care.

Lactation increases maternal nutritional demands, especially for energy, protein, omega-3 fatty acids, calcium, iodine, and vitamin D. These nutrients are critical not only for milk production and infant development but also for supporting maternal immune function and skin health [20]. For women with psoriasis, ensuring adequate intake of anti-inflammatory nutrients such as omega-3 s and antioxidants may help mitigate inflammation and reduce disease activity during the postpartum period. *Vitamin D*, in particular, warrants attention. Psoriatic patients often have suboptimal serum 25(OH)D levels, and both pregnancy and lactation further increase the need for vitamin D to support immune tolerance and bone health in the mother and infant. Supplementation may benefit psoriasis symptoms while also ensuring adequate transfer into breast milk [19].

Most topical therapies are considered safe during lactation, provided that they are not applied to areas where the infant may ingest the product (e.g., breast or nipple). However, systemic treatments require careful consideration. While some biologics (e.g., certolizumab pegol) demonstrate minimal transfer into breast milk and are considered low-risk, others have limited safety data and may require temporary discontinuation or avoidance [20, 21]. Shared decision-making between dermatologists, obstetricians, and lactation consultants is essential.

New mothers often face challenges such as sleep deprivation, altered dietary patterns, and limited time for self-care—all of which can exacerbate systemic inflammation and stress, potentially triggering psoriasis flares. Practical, evidence-based lifestyle support is especially valuable in this period [22].

- Encouraging simple, nutrient-dense meals (e.g., batch-prepared anti-inflammatory dishes)
- Supporting stress management with mindfulness techniques or postnatal support groups
- Promoting gentle, feasible forms of physical activity (e.g., walking and yoga)
- Addressing postpartum mood disorders, which are more prevalent in psoriatic patients and can worsen disease through psychoneuroimmune pathways

For specialist dermatologists, lactation presents an opportunity to reinforce lifestyle and nutritional counseling in the context of psoriasis. Optimizing maternal nutrition, minimizing inflammatory exposures (e.g., poor diet aad smoking), and safely navigating treatment decisions during breastfeeding can significantly improve maternal and infant outcomes.

11. Geriatric considerations in lifestyle and nutrition for psoriasis

Psoriasis in the elderly population presents unique challenges distinct from those encountered in younger adults. As global life expectancy rises, the prevalence of psoriasis among geriatric patients is increasing, necessitating tailored approaches to management. Aging is associated with physiological changes that influence skin integrity, immune function, nutritional status, and comorbidity profiles, all of which impact disease pathogenesis, progression, and treatment response. Lifestyle and nutritional factors are particularly critical in this age group, given the heightened vulnerability to both psoriasis complications and treatment-related adverse effects [23].

11.1 Age-related changes affecting psoriasis

Aging skin undergoes structural and functional alterations, including decreased epidermal thickness, reduced collagen synthesis, diminished barrier function, and impaired wound healing. These changes can modify the clinical presentation of psoriasis and may complicate topical and systemic treatment tolerance [24].

Immunosenescence, the gradual decline in immune competence with age, alters both innate and adaptive immunity. This may affect the inflammatory milieu in psoriasis, potentially leading to atypical disease patterns or altered flare dynamics. Additionally, chronic low-grade inflammation associated with aging ("inflammaging") can synergize with psoriatic inflammation, worsening disease severity or increasing comorbidity burden.

11.2 Nutritional challenges in the elderly with psoriasis

Malnutrition and micronutrient deficiencies are common in older adults due to factors such as reduced appetite, dental problems, altered taste, chronic illnesses, polypharmacy, and socioeconomic barriers. In psoriasis patients, these nutritional deficits may impair skin repair mechanisms and exacerbate systemic inflammation [25]. Adequate intake of protein, vitamins (particularly A, C, D, and E), zinc, and essential fatty acids is crucial for maintaining skin health and modulating immune responses. Vitamin D, in particular, plays a dual role in keratinocyte proliferation control and immune regulation, making deficiency a concern in elderly psoriatic patients. Furthermore, sarcopenia, or loss of muscle mass and strength, often seen in older adults, may be aggravated by chronic inflammation and sedentary lifestyle, negatively impacting physical function and quality of life [26].

11.3 Impact of comorbidities and polypharmacy

Geriatric patients with psoriasis frequently have multiple comorbid conditions such as cardiovascular disease, diabetes mellitus, hypertension, chronic kidney disease, and osteoarthritis. These comorbidities require careful consideration when recommending lifestyle interventions and nutritional strategies. Polypharmacy is also common in this population, increasing the risk of drug–nutrient interactions, adverse drug reactions, and medication non-adherence. For example, systemic psoriasis treatments may interact with medications used for comorbidities, and nutritional supplements can alter drug absorption or metabolism [27].

Pharmacologic treatment of psoriasis in geriatric patients requires careful balancing of efficacy and safety. Lifestyle and nutrition interventions serve as valuable adjuncts, potentially allowing for lower medication doses and minimizing adverse effects. Topical therapies may be preferred for localized disease, while systemic agents, including biologics, must be chosen with caution considering altered pharmacokinetics and polypharmacy risks. Nutritional status and lifestyle habits should be routinely assessed to optimize holistic care [17].

12. Clinical implications: Toward an integrative management model

Given the multifactorial nature of psoriasis, integrating lifestyle and nutrition into clinical care represents a pragmatic, evidence-based approach for improving outcomes. Dermatologists are well-positioned to initiate conversations about modifiable risk factors and deliver targeted guidance within a multidisciplinary framework.

Weight management should be a priority in overweight or obese patients, not only to reduce inflammation and improve skin symptoms but also to enhance the effectiveness of biologic agents. Even modest weight loss (5–10%) has been associated with meaningful improvements in PASI scores [18].

Nutritional counseling should emphasize the benefits of anti-inflammatory diets such as the Mediterranean pattern. Collaboration with registered dietitians can facilitate personalized meal planning and support behavioral change, especially in patients with complex dietary needs or comorbid metabolic disease [19].

Smoking cessation and *alcohol moderation* are critical but often under-addressed aspects of care. These behaviors can directly impair treatment response and increase cardiovascular risk. Dermatologists should routinely assess substance use and provide brief interventions, referring to addiction specialists when appropriate [20].

Stress management should be incorporated into comprehensive care, especially for patients with high disease burden, psychological comorbidity, or frequent flares. Referral to mental health professionals, structured CBT, or guided relaxation programs can offer substantial benefit [21].

Exercise prescriptions should be adapted to each patient's physical ability and preferences. Encouraging regular, moderate activity can improve both metabolic and psychological outcomes while supporting long-term disease control [22].

Ultimately, lifestyle medicine should be viewed not as ancillary but as integral to the long-term management of psoriasis. A patient-centered model—incorporating pharmacologic and non-pharmacologic strategies—offers the best opportunity for sustained remission, enhanced quality of life, and reduction of comorbid disease risk.

13. Future directions and research gaps

While lifestyle and nutritional interventions in psoriasis show significant promise, several critical knowledge gaps and methodological challenges remain. High-quality, large-scale randomized controlled trials (RCTs) are needed to establish causality and determine the most effective lifestyle strategies across different patient populations [23].

Standardization of dietary interventions remains a key limitation. Current studies use varied protocols, nutrient compositions, and outcome measures, making direct comparisons difficult. Future research should adopt standardized dietary assessment tools, nutrient biomarkers, and objective clinical endpoints such as PASI and Dermatology Life Quality Index (DLQI) [24].

Personalized nutrition is an emerging area of interest. Advances in nutrigenomics and metabolomics may help identify patient subgroups who respond more favorably to specific dietary patterns, enabling tailored interventions based on genetic, metabolic, or microbiome profiles [25].

In *pediatric populations*, data are especially scarce. Longitudinal studies are required to assess how early-life exposures, childhood diet, and psychosocial factors influence disease trajectory and long-term outcomes. Likewise, the safety and efficacy of interventions like intermittent fasting, ketogenic diets, or high-dose nutraceuticals in children remain poorly understood [26].

Another important direction involves the *gut-skin axis*. Preliminary findings suggest that probiotics, prebiotics, and microbiota-modulating diets may influence psoriasis, but robust clinical evidence is still lacking. Future trials should explore how microbiome alterations affect immune activity and therapeutic response [27].

Lastly, *implementation science* must be leveraged to translate existing evidence into real-world practice. Behavioral strategies, digital health tools, and multidisciplinary care models can help overcome adherence barriers and optimize lifestyle interventions in dermatology.

14. Conclusion

Psoriasis is a chronic inflammatory disease deeply influenced by lifestyle and nutritional factors. Evidence from clinical trials, mechanistic studies, and observational research consistently supports the role of diet, obesity, smoking, alcohol, stress, and physical activity in shaping disease severity, progression, and response to therapy.

For specialist dermatologists, integrating lifestyle medicine into clinical practice offers a powerful, low-risk complement to conventional treatment. Weight reduction, anti-inflammatory dietary patterns, smoking and alcohol cessation, stress management, and regular physical activity can significantly reduce inflammatory burden, improve skin and systemic symptoms, and enhance long-term outcomes.

Particular attention should be paid to pediatric patients and those with high-risk comorbidities, where early intervention may alter the disease trajectory and prevent complications. While further research is needed to refine recommendations and identify optimal strategies, existing evidence is sufficient to justify proactive lifestyle counseling as a core element of holistic psoriasis care.

As the field continues to evolve, dermatologists must take an active role in guiding patients through sustainable lifestyle change—empowering them not only to manage their skin but to optimize their overall health and well-being.

Author details

Shaimaa Farouk[1*], Rasha Aoun[2], Belal Muwafak[2], Hayder Al-Darraji[2] and Ammar Al-Dujaili[2]

1 Cairo Hospital of Dermatology and Venereology (Al Haud Al Marsoud), Egyptian Ministry of Health and Population, Cairo, Egypt

2 Egyptian Fellowship of Dermatology, Cairo, Egypt

*Address all correspondence to: dr.shaimaafarouk@gmail.com

References

[1] Naldi L, Chatenoud L, Linder D, et al. Cigarette smoking, body mass index, and stressful life events as risk factors for psoriasis: Results from an Italian case-control study. The Journal of Investigative Dermatology. 2005;**125**(1):61-67

[2] Jensen P, Zachariae C, Christensen R, et al. Effect of weight loss on the severity of psoriasis: A randomized clinical study. JAMA Dermatology. 2013;**149**(7):795-801

[3] Kyriakou A, Patsatsi A. Influence of obesity on psoriasis: A systematic review. Giornale Italiano di Dermatologia e Venereologia. 2018;**153**(3):326-335

[4] Coimbra S, Oliveira H, Reis F, et al. Interleukin (IL)-22, IL-17, and IL-23 levels in patients with psoriasis before and after treatment with etanercept and methotrexate. The British Journal of Dermatology. 2010;**163**(6):1282-1290

[5] Armstrong AW, Harskamp CT, Armstrong EJ. Psoriasis and metabolic syndrome: A systematic review and meta-analysis of observational studies. Journal of the American Academy of Dermatology. 2013;**68**(4):654-662

[6] Gisondi P, Del Giglio M, Girolomoni G. Weight loss improves the response of obese patients with moderate-to-severe chronic plaque psoriasis to low-dose cyclosporine therapy: A randomized controlled trial. The American Journal of Clinical Nutrition. 2008;**88**(5):1242-1247

[7] Debbaneh M, Millsop JW, Bhatia BK, et al. Diet and psoriasis, part II: Celiac disease and role of a gluten-free diet. Journal of the American Academy of Dermatology. 2014;**71**(2):350-358

[8] Barrea L, Balato N, Di Somma C, et al. Nutrition and psoriasis: Is there any association between the severity of the disease and adherence to the Mediterranean diet? Journal of Translational Medicine. 2015;**13**:18

[9] Upala S, Yong WC, Theparee T, Sanguankeo A. Effect of lifestyle weight loss intervention on disease severity in patients with psoriasis: A systematic review and meta-analysis. International Journal of Obesity. 2017;**41**(7):990-995

[10] Wolters M. Diet and psoriasis: Experimental data and clinical evidence. The British Journal of Dermatology. 2005;**153**(4):706-714

[11] Bhatia BK, Millsop JW, Debbaneh M, et al. Diet and psoriasis: Part I. Impact of weight loss interventions. Journal of the American Academy of Dermatology. 2014;**71**(1):133-140

[12] Zong H, Verma A, Rajagopalan S. Omega-3 fatty acids and cardiovascular outcomes: Systematic review and meta-analysis. Circulation. Cardiovascular Quality and Outcomes. 2016;**9**(5):560-568

[13] Simopoulos AP. The importance of the ratio of omega-6/omega-3 essential fatty acids. Biomedicine and Pharmacotherapy. 2002;**56**(8):365-379

[14] Wolk K, Mallbris L, Larsson P, et al. Excessive body weight and smoking associate with a high risk of onset of plaque psoriasis. Acta Dermato-Venereologica. 2009;**89**(5):492-497

[15] Addolorato G, Parente A, de Lorenzi G, et al. Rapid regression of psoriasis in a coeliac patient after gluten-free diet. Gut. 2003;**52**(4):514-517

[16] Setty AR, Curhan G, Choi HK. Obesity, waist circumference, weight change, and the risk of psoriasis in women: Nurses' health study II. Archives of Internal Medicine. 2007;**167**(15):1670-1675

[17] Addolorato G, Capristo E, Ghittoni G, et al. Anxiety and depression in psoriasis: A review. Journal of the European Academy of Dermatology and Venereology. 2005;**19**(2):205-213

[18] Henseler T, Christophers E. Disease concomitance in psoriasis. Journal of the American Academy of Dermatology. 1995;**32**(6):982-986

[19] Armstrong AW, Robertson AD, Wu J, et al. Undertreatment, treatment trends, and treatment dissatisfaction among patients with psoriasis and psoriatic arthritis in the United States. JAMA Dermatology. 2013;**149**(10):1180-1185

[20] Sampogna F, Tabolli S, Abeni D. Living with psoriasis: Prevalence of shame, anger, worry, and problems in daily activities and social life. Acta Dermato-Venereologica. 2012;**92**(3):299-303

[21] Arck PC, Slominski A, Theoharides TC, et al. Neuroimmunology of stress: Skin takes center stage. The Journal of Investigative Dermatology. 2006;**126**(8):1697-1704

[22] Richards HL, Fortune DG, Griffiths CE, Main CJ. The contribution of perceptions of stigmatisation to disability in patients with psoriasis. Journal of Psychosomatic Research. 2001;**50**(1):11-15

[23] Dalgard FJ, Gieler U, Tomas-Aragones L, et al. The psychological burden of skin diseases: A cross-sectional multicenter study among dermatological out-patients in 13 European countries. The Journal of Investigative Dermatology. 2015;**135**(4):984-991

[24] Reddy M, Martires K, Wu JJ. The role of diet in the treatment of psoriasis: A review. Cutis. 2013;**92**(3):149-152

[25] Balato N, Di Costanzo L, Patruno C, et al. Effect of weather and environmental factors on psoriasis. Journal of the European Academy of Dermatology and Venereology. 2013;**27**(10):1255-1262

[26] Boyd AS, Neldner KH. The isomorphic response of Koebner. International Journal of Dermatology. 1990;**29**(6):401-410

[27] Elmets CA, Leonardi CL, Davis DMR, et al. Joint AAD-NPF guidelines of care for the management and treatment of psoriasis with awareness and attention to comorbidities. Journal of the American Academy of Dermatology. 2019;**80**(4):1073-1113

Chapter 2

Flexibility of Biological Agents in the Treatment of Psoriasis

Muhammed Ali Mergen, Tubanur Çetinarslan and Aylin Türel Ermertcan

Abstract

Psoriasis represents a chronic inflammatory condition driven by immune dysregulation, manifesting with systemic and cutaneous features. It affects both children and adults, involving skin, nails, and joints. While commonly seen on the scalp and extensor areas such as the elbows and knees, it may also involve more challenging sites including the face, genital region, and palmoplantar areas. Psoriasis is associated with various comorbidities including psoriatic arthritis, obesity, metabolic syndrome, hypertension, diabetes, cardiovascular diseases, inflammatory bowel disease, severe infections, and other autoimmune conditions. According to the latest European guidelines, biological therapies are recommended for patients with moderate-to-severe psoriasis when topical or systemic conventional treatments fail to provide adequate disease control or cause significant adverse effects. The choice of biologic is influenced by many factors such as clinical subtype, comorbidities, site of involvement and need for intermittent treatment. Assessment of treatment response during the induction and maintenance phases is essential in determining the continuation or modification of therapy. However, there are no universally accepted guidelines regarding dose escalation, interval shortening strategies, switching between biologics, treatment interruption or discontinuation, and the challenges encountered upon re-initiation. This review aims to offer practical insights into these aspects, based on data from multicenter randomized controlled trials, systematic reviews, meta-analyses, and current treatment guidelines.

Keywords: psoriasis, biologics, flexibility, switching, dose adjustment

1. Introduction

Psoriasis is a chronic inflammatory condition of autoimmune origin, with systemic involvement, affecting nearly 125 million people worldwide [1]. It can occur at any age, with peak onset between 30–39 and 50–69 years [2]. The most common subtype is chronic plaque psoriasis, but other forms such as guttate, pustular, and erythrodermic psoriasis may also occur [3]. In addition to the typical involvement of the scalp, elbows, and knees, psoriasis can also affect difficult-to-treat areas including the nails, face, genital region, and palmoplantar surfaces [3]. Beyond its cutaneous manifestations, psoriasis is increasingly recognized as a multi-system condition with a range of associated comorbidities [4]. These include psoriatic arthritis, obesity, metabolic syndrome, hypertension, diabetes, cardiovascular disease, inflammatory bowel disease, malignancies, autoimmune conditions, and increased susceptibility to serious infections [4]. The presence of these comorbidities complicates clinical decision-making and influences both prognosis and long-term treatment outcomes [4].

According to the latest European guidelines, conventional systemic agents such as methotrexate, acitretin, fumarates, and cyclosporine, are recommended as first-line therapies for patients with moderate-to-severe psoriasis. However, in cases where these treatments fail to achieve adequate disease control, are contraindicated, or result in significant adverse effects, biologic therapies targeting pivotal cytokines in psoriasis pathogenesis, particularly tumor necrosis factor-alpha (TNF-α), interleukin (IL)-12/23, IL-17, and IL-23, are advised [5]. Biologic agents demonstrate higher clinical efficacy and comparable or superior safety profiles than systemic conventional therapies and offer the added advantage of targeted action and improved patient adherence [6, 7]. Despite the advances in biologic treatment, clinical practice often requires flexibility in the application of these agents. Issues such as partial response, secondary loss of efficacy, patient-specific comorbidities, and the need for treatment interruption (e.g., due to infections, surgery, or pregnancy) necessitate individualized treatment strategies [5, 8]. Unfortunately, current guidelines offer limited direction on practical considerations such as dose escalation, interval shortening, switching between biologics, treatment interruption, and re-initiation protocols [5, 8].

The aim of this review is to provide an evidence-based overview of flexibility strategies in the use of biologic agents for psoriasis, based on randomized controlled trials, systematic reviews, real-world studies, and international guidelines.

2. Psoriasis and comorbidities

Psoriasis is a multi-systemic inflammatory disease associated with a wide range of comorbidities that influence therapeutic decisions and prognosis [4]. These comorbidities often share overlapping immunopathogenic mechanisms, particularly involving TNF-α, IL-17, and IL-23 pathways [4]. In this section, the most common comorbidities observed in patients with psoriasis and which biologic agents are preferred or should be avoided in the presence of each are discussed.

2.1 Comorbidities

2.1.1 Psoriatic arthritis (PsA)

Psoriatic arthritis (PsA) is an immune-mediated joint disease that involves peripheral and axial joints as well as entheses and commonly coexists with skin and nail involvement [9]. It occurs in approximately 6–42% of patients with psoriasis, and its prevalence increases with the severity and duration of skin disease [4]. Cutaneous involvement typically precedes joint symptoms, though PsA may remain undiagnosed in up to 15.5% of psoriasis patients at the time of presentation [10]. Early recognition is important to prevent irreversible joint damage and disability [10].

Several screening tools such as Psoriasis Epidemiology Screening Tool (PEST), Psoriasis and Arthritis Screening Questionnaire (PASQ), and the Classification Criteria for Psoriatic Arthritis (CASPAR) criteria have been developed to assist diagnosis [11]. Although the CASPAR criteria demonstrate high specificity (99.1%), their relatively lower sensitivity (approximately 87.4%) limits their utility in detecting early-stage PsA [11].

Enhanced interdisciplinary collaboration and use of simplified mnemonics like "PSA" (Pain, Stiffness/Sausage digit, Axial involvement) may facilitate earlier identification [12].

Patients with comorbid PsA report greater impairment in physical function, higher prevalence of cardiovascular and metabolic comorbidities, and reduced quality of life compared to psoriasis-only patients [13, 14]. Initiating treatment without delay in patients with psoriatic arthritis plays a crucial role in preserving joint function and limiting irreversible structural damage. Delays over 6 months are associated with worse Health Assessment Questionnaire (HAQ) scores and joint erosions [15, 16]. Moreover, PsA often leads to work disability and productivity loss, which can be mitigated by effective treatment [15, 16]. Biologic therapies tailored to both skin and joint involvement have demonstrated efficacy in improving disease activity and patient-reported outcomes, especially when initiated early [16, 17].

2.1.2 Cardiovascular disease (CVD)

Psoriasis has been linked to a higher burden of cardiovascular risk factors, notably type 2 diabetes, hypertension, dyslipidemia, and obesity [18]. A significantly higher prevalence of metabolic syndrome has been observed in both adult and pediatric psoriasis populations [4]. Beyond conventional risk factors, psoriasis is linked to vascular inflammation. Studies utilizing fluorodeoxyglucose F-18 positron emission tomography-computed tomography (FDG PET/CT) imaging have demonstrated increased aortic vascular inflammation and coronary plaque burden in patients with psoriasis [19]. Improvements in skin disease severity correlate with reduced vascular inflammation over time, suggesting a systemic inflammatory contribution to cardiovascular risk [20]. Furthermore, longer psoriasis duration has been associated with an increased risk of major adverse cardiovascular events (MACE), highlighting the importance of cumulative inflammatory exposure [21].

Treatment with tumor necrosis factor inhibitors (TNFi) has been associated with reductions in inflammatory markers such as C-reactive protein (CRP) [22]. Retrospective cohort studies have demonstrated a lower risk of MACE in psoriasis patients treated with TNFi compared to those on methotrexate, phototherapy, or topical agents [23–25]. Moreover, biologic therapy (adalimumab, etanercept, infliximab and ustekinumab) may attenuate the progression of coronary artery disease, as shown by coronary CT angiography over a 13-month period in patients with severe psoriasis [26].

However, not all findings are consistent. Randomized controlled trials (RCTs) using FDG PET/CT have shown no significant reduction in vascular inflammation after TNFi therapy compared to placebo [27, 28]. Thus, while observational data suggest a cardioprotective effect of biologics in ischemic heart diseases, particularly TNF inhibitors, RCTs have yielded mixed results, and the true impact on cardiovascular risk remains under investigation.

2.1.3 Obesity and metabolic syndrome

Obesity has been consistently identified as an independent contributor to the risk of developing psoriasis. Multiple cohort studies have indicated that there is a positive correlation between higher body mass index (BMI) and incidence of psoriasis [29]. A meta-analysis reported an odds ratio (OR) of 1.66 for the association between psoriasis and obesity [30]. When stratified by disease severity, OR for obesity in patients with mild psoriasis was 1.46, and for severe psoriasis, 2.23 [30].

Metabolic syndrome is defined as the coexistence of central obesity, hypertension, insulin resistance, and dyslipidemia [31]. Multiple studies have demonstrated that both metabolic syndrome and its individual components are significantly more prevalent among patients with psoriasis compared to the general population [31]. A meta-analysis reported an OR of 2.26 for the association between psoriasis and metabolic syndrome [31].

Supporting these findings, a cross-sectional study by Langan et al. in the UK demonstrated a dose-dependent relationship between psoriasis severity and both obesity and the risk of metabolic syndrome [32]. These results suggest that both the onset and severity of psoriasis are positively associated with increasing levels of obesity and highlight the importance of weight management in the overall care of psoriasis patients.

2.1.4 Inflammatory bowel disease (IBD)

Psoriasis and inflammatory bowel diseases (IBD), including Crohn's disease (CD) and ulcerative colitis (UC), appear to share overlapping genetic and immunological mechanisms [4]. While the precise epidemiological relationship between these conditions remains unclear, numerous studies have reported a higher prevalence and incidence of IBD in individuals with psoriasis [33, 34]. Evidences suggest a stronger association between psoriasis and CD than with UC [33, 34].

2.1.5 Psychological comorbidities

Patients with psoriasis are more likely to experience depression compared to the general population [35]. Emerging data indicate that comorbid major depressive disorder (MDD) further compounds other disease risks. In a prospective cohort study, psoriasis patients with MDD were significantly more prone to develop psoriatic arthritis than those without depression [36]. Moreover, studies showed that concurrent depression in psoriasis correlated with elevated rates of myocardial infarction, stroke, cardiovascular mortality, and greater vascular inflammation [37, 38].

In addition to depression, anxiety disorders and suicidal thoughts are more prevalent among psoriasis patients compared to the general population [39, 40]. These findings highlight the critical need for routine screening and integrated treatment of mental health conditions in the comprehensive care of psoriasis patients.

2.1.6 Other comorbidities

Individuals with psoriasis demonstrate a higher prevalence of mild liver diseases as well as chronic kidney disease when compared to the general population [4]. Moreover, the risk of malignancies, especially cutaneous T cell lymphoma, and serious infections appears to be elevated in patients with psoriasis [4]. Recently, pulmonary diseases such as chronic obstructive pulmonary disease and obstructive sleep apnea have also been increasingly recognized as part of the psoriasis-associated systemic disease burden [4].

2.2 Biologic selection according to comorbidities

The presence of comorbidities significantly influences the choice of biologic agent. Clinical guidelines and expert consensus recommend tailoring treatment based on individual risk profiles, as outlined in **Table 1** [5, 41]:

Comorbidity	Preferred biologics	To avoid
PsA*	1. TNF-alfa-i, secukinumab, ixekizumab, IL-23-i 2. Brodalumab, bimekizumab, apremilast 3. Tildrakizumab, ustekinumab, deucravacitinib	
Obesity**	1. IL-17-i, ustekinumab 2. IL-23-i, apremilast 3. TNF-alfa-i	
Advanced heart failure	1. IL-17-i, IL-23-i 2. Ustekinumab	TNF-alfa-i in severe heart failure (NYHA III-IV)
İschemic heart disease	1. TNF-alfa-i 2. IL-17-i, IL-23-i, apremilast 3. Ustekinumab	
Depression/ suicidality	1. IL-23-i 2. Secukinumab, ixekizumab, ustekinumab 3. TNF-alfa-i	Brodalumab and apremilast
IBD	1. Adalimumab, infliximab 2. Ustekinumab, certolizumab pegol, IL-23-i 3. Apremilast	IL-17-i
Multiple sclerosis	1. IL-17-i 2. Ustekinumab 3. IL-23-i	TNF-alfa-i
Malignancy history	1. IL-17-i, IL-23-i 2. Ustekinumab	TNF-alfa-i
Pregnancy/lactation	1. Certolizumab pegol	Most other biologics

PsA, psoriatic arthritis; IL, interleukin; TNF, tumor necrosis factor; CVD, cardiovascular diseases; IBD, inflammatory bowel disease; NYHA, New York Heart Association.
**TNF-α inhibitors and IL-17-i are firstly recommended in axial spondylarthritis or enthesitis.*
***Weight-based dosing is recommended for ustekinumab, and TNF-α inhibitors may require dose adjustments in patients with high body mass index.*

Table 1.
Overview of biological therapy options in most common comorbidities.

3. Assessment of treatment response

Evaluating treatment response in psoriasis is essential to ensure therapeutic success and guide ongoing management [42]. The most widely used metrics in both clinical trials and daily practice are the Psoriasis Area and Severity Index (PASI) and the Dermatology Life Quality Index (DLQI) [42, 43]. The induction phase refers to the initial stage of biologic treatment, typically lasting up to week 16. However, depending on the specific agent and dosing schedule, this period may be extended up to week 24, based on clinical judgment [44]. The maintenance phase begins following the completion of the induction period and represents the ongoing treatment phase. During this period, therapeutic effectiveness should be evaluated at regular intervals in line with current clinical guidelines [44].

3.1 Treatment goals in induction and maintenance phases

Achievement of a ≥75% reduction in PASI score from baseline at the end of the induction phase is considered treatment success. In such cases, continuation of the current therapeutic regimen is recommended [44, 45]. Failure to reach at least a 50%

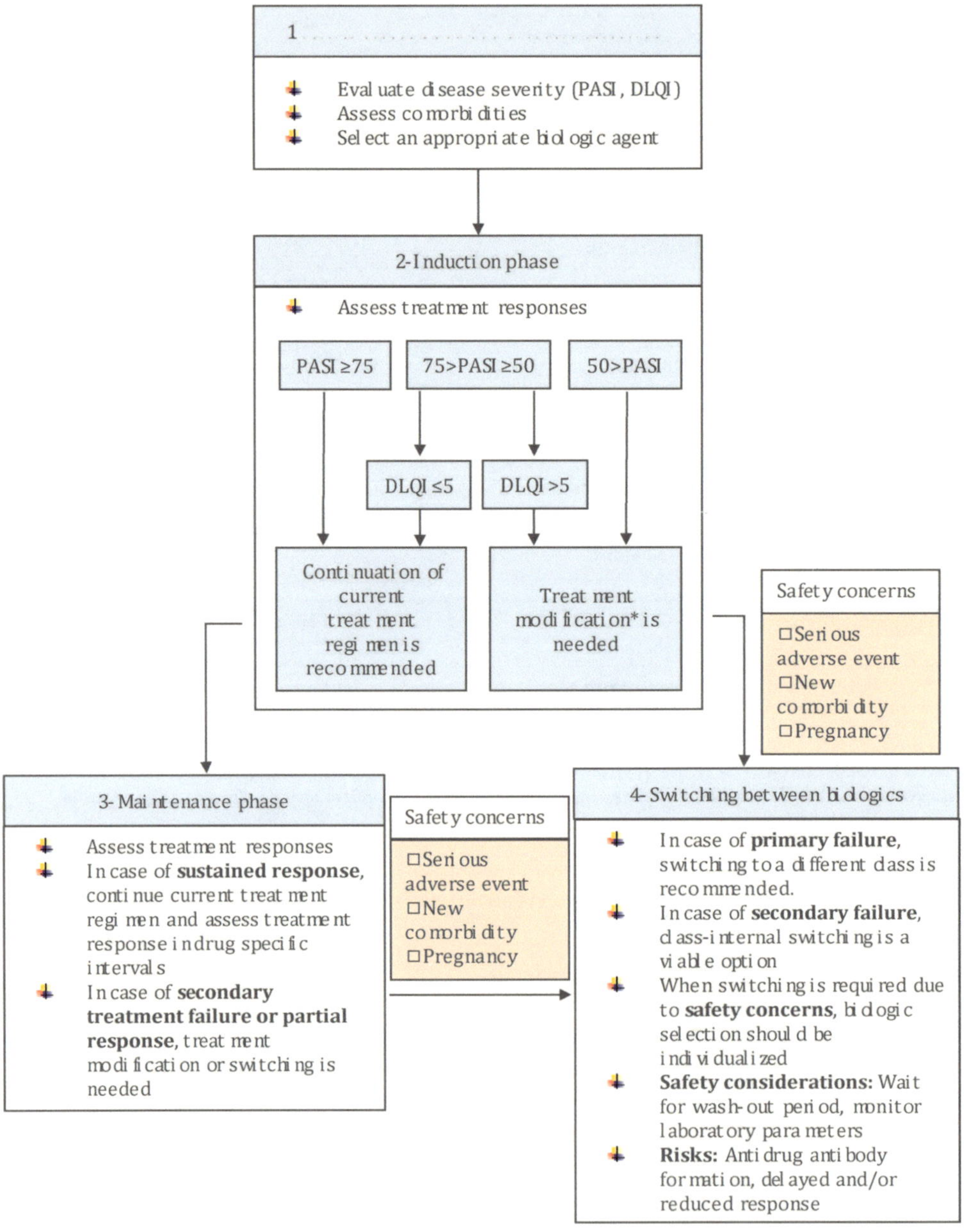

Figure 1.
*Biologic therapy algorithm for induction, maintenance and switching. PASI, Psoriasis Area and Severity Index; DLQI, Dermatology Life Quality Index. *Treatment modification strategies are dose escalation, interval shortening, addition of adjunctive therapies, optimization of adjunctive therapies (e.g., switch from oral to subcutaneous), inpatient application of adjunctive therapies, and management of modifiable factors contributing to poor response (e.g., obesity and poor compliance).*

improvement in PASI score during the induction period is interpreted as primary treatment failure, for which modification of the therapeutic approach is advised [44, 45]. When PASI improvement ranges between 50% and 74%, treatment decisions should be guided by the patient's quality of life. If the DLQI remains above 5 or shows no significant improvement, adjustment of the treatment regimen is appropriate. Conversely, in patients who report a DLQI of 5 or less, the existing therapy may be maintained [44, 45].

A sustained PASI improvement of at least 75% from baseline during the maintenance period is accepted as a successful long-term therapeutic outcome. In such cases, continuation of the current biologic regimen is recommended [44]. When PASI improvement falls below 50% during maintenance therapy, this is interpreted as secondary treatment failure. In these patients, it is advisable to revise the therapeutic strategy, such as by switching agents or adjusting the regimen [44, 45].

In patients with sustained PASI improvement between 50% and 74%, DLQI plays a decisive role in clinical decision-making. If the DLQI score remains above 5 or shows no meaningful improvement, treatment adjustment is warranted. Conversely, if DLQI is maintained at ≤5, continuation of the existing therapy is considered appropriate [44, 45].

Treatment decisions in biologic therapy require systematic evaluation of both clinical response and individual patient factors. The algorithm presented in **Figure 1** summarizes the overall approach to induction, maintenance, and switching strategies, integrating PASI and DLQI thresholds, clinical phase-specific definitions of success or failure, and flexibility considerations such as dose adjustments or class switching [5, 44, 45].

4. Treatment modification strategies in biologic therapy

Dose escalation or interval shortening may be considered in patients with suboptimal response, particularly in cases of obesity, disease relapse within the dosing interval, or suspected subtherapeutic drug levels. However, such adjustments may increase the risk of adverse events [45]. Dose escalation and interval shortening strategies are summarized in **Table 2** [45–50].

In cases of a partial response or disease flare during biologic therapy, adjunctive treatments may be considered to enhance therapeutic efficacy without switching the primary biologic agent [8, 51]. The addition of topical corticosteroids with or without combination with retinoids, vitamin D analogs or topical calcineurin inhibitors can be effective in controlling recalcitrant lesions, particularly in difficult-to-treat anatomical regions [8, 51–54]. This strategy may be beneficial for the maintenance of initial responses, improvement of efficacy in partial responders and mitigation of localized flare-ups during maintenance [52]. Moreover, adjunctive therapy may act as a temporary measure to delay or avoid premature switching, dose escalation, or interval shortening [52]. Although there is no formal approval for combining biologic agents with systemic conventional therapies in psoriasis, combinations with acitretin may improve clinical efficacy and combinations with methotrexate may reduce immunogenicity, thus providing long-term disease control [8]. However, combinations with cyclosporine are not suitable in terms of safety [8]. It is also important to be aware of an increased risk of infection with such combinations [5]. Similar to systemic conventional therapies, adjunctive use of phototherapy with biological therapies increases efficacy [8]. However, the long-term safety profile of such combinations remains uncertain due to the lack of randomized controlled trials [8].

Biologic agent	Standard dosing regimen	Suggested dose escalation/interval shortening strategy
Adalimumab	40 mg every other week	40 mg per week
Etanercept	50 mg per week	50 mg twice weekly
Infliximab*	5 mg/kg every 8 weeks	5 mg/kg every 6 weeks
Certolizumab pegol	200 mg every other week	400 mg every other week
Ustekinumab* ≤100 kg >100 kg	45 mg every 12 weeks 90 mg every 12 weeks	90 mg every 8–12 weeks 90 mg every 8 weeks
Ixekizumab*	80 mg every 4 weeks	80 mg every 2 weeks
Tildrakizumab	100 mg every 12 weeks	200 mg every 12 weeks
Secukinumab	300 mg every 4 weeks	300 mg every 2 weeks
Bimekizumab	320 mg every 8 weeks	320 mg every 4 weeks
Risankizumab**	150 mg every 12 weeks	150 mg every 8 weeks
Guselkumab**	100 mg every 8 weeks	100 mg every 4–6 weeks

**Off-license use.*
***To date, no prospective studies have evaluated dose escalation or interval-shortening strategies for risankizumab and guselkumab. Current knowledge is primarily based on real-world observations and expert opinion. The rate of dose escalation with risankizumab has been reported to be approximately 2%, suggesting that the need for dose adjustment is rare due to the drug's high efficacy and long half-life.*

Table 2.
Dose escalation and interval shortening strategies.

All parameters recommended for monitoring when used as monotherapy for biologic agents should also be considered for combination therapy with conventional systemic therapies [8]. The overall monitoring interval should be guided according to the drug requiring the most stringent monitoring [8]. If there is a potential for synergistic toxicity, closer monitoring may be warranted, and additional laboratory assessments may be necessary [8]. Conventional systemic therapy should be added starting with the lowest effective dose, for example, 5–10 mg/week methotrexate, to minimize adverse effects while assessing tolerability [8].

Combination regimens involving etanercept with methotrexate or etanercept with acitretin have been shown to enhance therapeutic efficacy without introducing significant additional toxicity, making them viable options in clinical practice [55, 56]. Although there is no randomized clinical trial investigating the concurrent use of infliximab and methotrexate in psoriasis, existing evidence suggests that the addition of low-dose methotrexate may reduce the development of anti-drug antibodies against infliximab [5]. This immunomodulatory effect helps preserve drug efficacy and may reduce the risk of secondary treatment failure [5].

The combination of adalimumab or ustekinumab with methotrexate has been shown to enhance clinical efficacy in patients with psoriasis [57]. While the evidence supporting combination strategies involving IL-17 or IL-23 inhibitors remains limited, current data do not indicate any major safety concerns with these regimens [8, 58]. Registry-based studies have suggested that patients undergoing combination therapy are more likely to have concomitant psoriatic arthritis (PsA). However, it is important to note that adverse events—particularly those related to safety—appear to be more frequent with combination regimens compared to biologic monotherapy [58, 59]. Treatment combinations in psoriasis are summarized in **Table 3** [5, 60].

	Cyclosporine	Methotrexate	Acitretin	Phototherapy
Adalimumab*	–	+	+	+
Etanercept*	–	+	+	+
Infliximab	–	+	+	–
Ustekinumab	–	+	?	?
IL-17 i**	?	?	?	?
IL-23 i**	?	?	?	?

+/– combination is useful/not useful, ? insufficient data.
**There are studies showing that the combination of etanercept or adalimumab with narrowband UVB increase the clinical efficacy, their combination with PUVA is not recommended due to the risk of phototoxicity.*
***While the evidence supporting combination strategies involving IL-17 or IL-23 inhibitors remains limited, current data do not indicate any major safety concerns with these regimens.*

Table 3.
Possible combinations of biologics with systemic conventional therapies and phototherapy in psoriasis.

5. Switching between biologic agents: Strategies and current evidence

5.1 Indications for switching biologic therapy

Switching biologic agents should be considered for patients with psoriasis experiencing safety concerns (e.g., serious adverse event and pregnancy), a lack of adequate response despite modification strategies or development of new comorbidities [5, 45, 61]. Real-world analyses from 2018 to 2022 show that 14.4% of patients switch biologics within 1 year of initiation and 26% of patients switch within 2 years [62]. This study has shown that IL-23 inhibitors have the lowest rates of switching (6.4% at 12 months and 12.7% at 24 months) [62]. TNF inhibitors have the highest switch rates of 24.8% at 12 months and 39.1% at 24 months [62]. While 35.2% of those who switched preferred IL-17 inhibitors, 37.4% of those who switched preferred IL-23 inhibitors [62]. The biologic with the lowest switch rate is risankizumab, followed by guselkumab [62]. Being bio-experienced, aging and being female are predictors of switching in patients with psoriasis receiving biologic therapies [62].

In the context of switching due to insufficient clinical response, the therapeutic effect of the subsequent biologic may be diminished compared to biologic-naive patients [5, 63]. Therefore, switching to an agent from a different class is generally favored in case of primary treatment failures [5, 63]. However, in cases of secondary treatment failure or partial responses, class-internal switching is a viable and effective approach [5, 63]. There is no consensus on the necessity of a washout period between biologic agents [5, 63]. Some recommendations suggest a gap of at least 1 month or one complete dosing cycle is recommended before switching to a new biologic agent [5, 45, 63]. Nevertheless, evidence indicates that switching to a new therapy at standard maintenance doses without a washout does not negatively impact treatment outcomes [5, 63]. Real-world data support effective switching from IL-17 inhibitors to anti-TNF or ustekinumab in patients with inadequate response [5, 63]. Furthermore, IL-17 and IL-23 inhibitors have demonstrated favorable outcomes in patients who previously failed to respond to TNF-α inhibitors or ustekinumab [5, 8, 63]. While current data on transitions between IL-17 and IL-23 inhibitors remain limited, class-internal switching following IL-17 inhibitor failure has yielded promising results in clinical practice [63]. A real-life 16-week retrospective study has shown that a majority of patients with inadequate responses to IL-17 and IL-12/23 inhibitors achieved near-complete skin clearance after switching to risankizumab [64].

Safety concerns associated with biologic therapies may be universal across agents or may vary depending on the specific drug or its molecular class [63]. For instance, anti-TNF agents have been linked to adverse events such as tuberculosis, congestive heart failure, demyelinating disorders (e.g., multiple sclerosis), and drug-induced lupus erythematosus, whereas IL-17 inhibitors are more commonly associated with mucocutaneous candidiasis and exacerbation or induction of inflammatory bowel disease [5, 63, 65]. In cases of TNFi-related safety concerns, IL-17 or IL-23 inhibitors are often preferred alternatives [63]. Similarly, if adverse events occur with IL-17 inhibitors, TNFi or IL-23 inhibitors may be appropriate [63]. Ustekinumab is particularly favored when lupus-like reactions develop during anti-TNF or IL-17 therapy. If the lupus-like reaction arises with a TNF inhibitor, switching to another TNFi agent may still be considered under close clinical monitoring [65, 66]. When paradoxical reactions necessitate discontinuation, switching to a biologic with a different molecular target is advised due to the potential class effect involved [63]. Conversely, adverse events such as alopecia areata are believed to be drug-specific and may not recur with another agent from the same class [63]. When switching is required due to safety concerns, biological agent from a different class is preferred, and a drug-free period may be required until safety parameters return to normal or become stable [61]. In the WHO pharmacovigilance study, certolizumab pegol was highlighted as a safe option during pregnancy. By contrast, there is insufficient data for IL-17 and IL-23 inhibitors [67].

Clinical studies show that switching from etanercept to adalimumab does not result in reduced treatment efficacy, even when the former therapy was ineffective [47]. However, switching from adalimumab to etanercept following primary failure may yield less favorable results. In contrast, switching due to secondary failure tends to be associated with improved outcomes [47]. Positive outcomes have also been reported in patients switched from TNFi to ustekinumab due to inadequate response, though the magnitude of benefit may be attenuated [47]. Likewise, in patients switched to secukinumab, reduced response rates were observed among those with previous biologic failure. However, higher dosing (e.g., 300 mg) of secukinumab and more frequent administration of ixekizumab (e.g., every other week) has been associated with improved PASI responses in these patients [47]. Additionally, switching to guselkumab or risankizumab after the failure of previous biologics has shown significant clinical benefit [47].

6. Dose reduction and discontinuation of biologic therapy

6.1 TNF-α inhibitors

There is growing evidence that carefully selected patients in stable remission can undergo dose tapering, usually by extending intervals with maintained disease control [68, 69]. In a randomized clinical trial, intervals of adalimumab or etanercept were prolonged to 67% and then 50% of the standard dose in stepwise. Half of patients successfully maintain low disease activity over 1 year [69]. However, the dose-reduction group had a slight increase in median PASI compared to usual dosing [69]. No increase in serious adverse events was seen, and quality-of-life outcomes remained comparable [69]. These findings suggest that gradual interval extension can be attempted in patients with durable minimal disease, with close monitoring for flare [69]. Patients must be counseled that any signs of loss of response warrant re-escalation to the full dose to prevent significant relapse [69].

Continuous therapy is generally more effective in sustaining remission than interrupted therapy. Withdrawal of TNF inhibitors often leads to prompt recurrence of psoriasis activity [70]. In fact, systematic reviews indicate that full discontinuation of TNF inhibitors typically results in relapse within a median of 3 to 4 months [71]. Nearly all patients eventually relapse if the drug is stopped: in one cohort, more than 90% of patients relapsed within 2 years after stopping a TNF or ustekinumab [72]. Therefore, maintaining a reduced dosing schedule may delay or prevent relapse. While dose reduction can preserve long-term efficacy for many patients, complete withdrawal can lead to significantly higher flare rates. Patients considered for tapering should be those with sustained skin clearance or low disease activity for at least 1 year, no recent flares, and no active PsA or any other comorbidity [61].

Intermittent dosing of TNF inhibitors can increase the risk of anti-drug antibody (ADA) formation, potentially reducing drug efficacy upon re-exposure. This is especially true for infliximab whose intermittent dosing led to high ADA rates and infusion reactions in RCTs [70]. Etanercept and adalimumab also carry a risk of ADA development, though a bit lower than infliximab [70]. Withdrawal of TNF inhibitors has a higher risk of ADA because continuous therapy minimizes immunogenicity and maintains efficacy [70]. Thus, complete discontinuation is generally not recommended in routine practice unless there is pregnancy, serious adverse event, or patient request. Most guidelines favor dose reduction over complete cessation [70].

If re-initiation is needed after cessation, resuming the usual maintenance dosing with close monitoring is advised in short interruptions. Whereas a re-induction regimen is needed in long interruptions [70].

6.2 IL-12/23 inhibitor

Long dosing interval makes ustekinumab a candidate for cautious interval extension in stable patients. In a randomized clinical trial, patients receiving ustekinumab treatment at usual intervals were compared with patients who underwent an interval extension strategy [69]. Fifty-three percent of patients were able to maintain low disease activity in the dose-reduction group [69]. However, the other half required reversion to the usual interval due to psoriasis worsening [69]. Similar to TNF inhibitors, dose reduction should be attempted only in very stable patients.

An 8-year multicenter study has shown that the median time to relapse after discontinuation of ustekinumab is 4 to 5 months. Long-term observations have shown that nearly all patients relapsed within 36 months [73]. Therefore, complete discontinuation should be reserved for conditions like pregnancy, severe infection, or patient requests.

In a 52-week double-blind randomized controlled trial, ADA to ustekinumab has been reported in 5.4% of patients [74]. There is no known randomized clinical study comparing the ADA titers in patients receiving ustekinumab at usual intervals with ones receiving at extended intervals. Yet, no major safety signals have emerged from dose reduction studies. Tapering did not lead to increased adverse events or inflammatory reactions. This indicates that from a safety standpoint, spacing out doses is not harmful; the main risk is loss of efficacy [69, 70].

In a 76-week double-blind, randomized controlled trial, re-initiation for the withdrawal group was started after the loss of PASI 75 response [75]. About 85.6% of patients recaptured response within 3 months [75]. However, retreatment efficacy did not reach the original heights in most biologics. Thus, continuous long-term therapy remains the preferred strategy for persistent control [72, 73].

6.3 IL-17 inhibitors

IL-17 inhibitors typically require uninterrupted dosing to sustain remission because their mechanism and pharmacokinetics favor regular administration. In a double-blind, randomized controlled trial, patients who achieved a 75% response at week 12 were re-randomized as receiving treatment as needed or receiving treatment with usual intervals [76]. While 78.2% of patients receiving at usual intervals maintained a PASI 75 response, 67.7% of patients receiving retreatment as needed maintained a PASI 75 response [76]. ADA development to secukinumab and safety profiles were similar in between groups [76]. On a positive note, IL-17 inhibitors tend to have low immunogenicity, which aids in successful retreatment.

A systematic review has shown that IL-17 inhibitor discontinuation was associated with shorter median remission durations (about 2–6 months) than IL-23 inhibitors (about 5–10 months) [71]. In a double-blind withdrawal study, patients who achieved minimal disease activity were re-randomized as a withdrawal treatment group and continued treatment group [77]. While 85% of patients experienced relapse in the withdrawal treatment group, 38% of patients experienced relapse in the continued treatment group [77]. Thus, routine discontinuation of IL-17 inhibitors is discouraged unless there are conditions like pregnancy, serious infection or patient request. In the study, 96% of patients recaptured response within a month after re-initiation for the patients who experienced relapse [77]. In conclusion, spacing out doses or withdrawal is not recommended. Fortunately, in cases where the treatment needs to be interrupted or stopped when the cause is eliminated and treatment is re-initiated, the responses can be achieved in a short time.

6.4 IL-23 inhibitors

Recent studies highlight the potential for dose interval extension in patients receiving IL-23 inhibitors [78]. Phase 3b GUIDE trial investigated guselkumab in patients who achieved PASI 100 response within 6 months [78]. Participants were randomized to maintain the standard 8-week regimen or transition to a 16-week schedule [79]. Findings indicated that extended dosing maintained efficacy, with over 90% of patients in both groups sustaining near-complete skin clearance at week 68, demonstrating non-inferiority of the extended interval [78]. Similar interval modifications are being explored for risankizumab, although current evidence remains largely anecdotal [71]. Therefore, IL-23 inhibitors may be promising candidates for tailored de-escalation strategies in the management of psoriasis [71].

IL-23 inhibitors have demonstrated the most prolonged maintenance of psoriasis remission following treatment cessation among all biologic classes [71]. In studies involving guselkumab, the median time to relapse was approximately 23 weeks after the last dose [80]. Similarly, risankizumab has shown a median relapse time of about 42 weeks post-treatment, reflecting sustained efficacy even after discontinuation [71, 81]. This makes IL-23 inhibitors particularly suitable for situations where a planned drug-free period is necessary, such as surgery, pregnancy, or temporary contraindications. Despite their prolonged effect, most patients eventually relapse within a year of discontinuation [72]. Real-world evidence confirms that the majority of patients restart systemic therapy within 12 months [72].

IL-23 inhibitors are associated with low immunogenicity profiles [82]. While the incidence of ADA formation with guselkumab ranged from 4.1% to 14.7%, the incidence of neutralizing antibodies ranged from 0.1% to 0.6%. Risankizumab showed a higher frequency of ADA development, with reported rates between 14% and 31%, though neutralizing antibodies occur in 2.4–16% of cases [82]. Most antibodies tend to be of low titer and do not meaningfully impact therapeutic efficacy [82].

A small subset of psoriasis patients may sustain remission after discontinuation of IL-23 inhibitors, particularly with those achieving PASI90 responses within 12 weeks [80]. Favorable predictors include biologic-naive status, lower BMI, and shorter disease duration [80].

IL-23 inhibitors allow for effective retreatment after therapy interruption, with most patients regaining previous levels of clearance upon re-initiation [83]. In VOYAGE 2 study, following discontinuation of guselkumab, 80.4% of patients who lost their PASI-90 response and were restarted recaptured response at week 20 [83]. Even after long drug-free periods, response is typically recaptured without added safety concerns. This supports a flexible treatment model where temporary discontinuation is feasible when clinically necessary.

7. Conclusion

Psoriasis is a chronic inflammatory condition with systemic involvement. Its management often requires a flexible, patient-centered approach in order to maximize the benefits of biological therapies. It is associated with a wide range of comorbidities such as PsA, CVD, obesity, metabolic syndrome, IBD, depression, and suicidality. The presence of comorbidities significantly influences the choice of biologic agent. Therefore, severity and comorbidity evaluation is important in the initial assessment and choice of biological therapy.

In case of a lack of adequate response, treatment modification strategies such as dose escalation, interval shortening or addition of adjunctive treatments are needed. Combination of biologic agents with topical and systemic conventional therapies may be beneficial for the maintenance of initial responses, improvement of efficacy in partial responders, mitigation of localized flare-ups during maintenance and decreasing anti-drug antibody levels. Additionally, it may act as a temporary measure to delay or avoid premature switching.

Switching biologic agents should be considered for patients with psoriasis experiencing safety concerns (e.g., serious adverse event and pregnancy), a lack of adequate response despite modification strategies or development of new comorbidities. Being bio-experienced, aging and being female are predictors of switching in patients with psoriasis receiving biologic therapies. While switching to an agent from a different class is generally favored in case of primary treatment failures, class-internal switching is a viable and effective approach in cases of secondary treatment failure or partial responses.

While a drug-free period is needed in case of switching due to safety concerns, a gap of 1 month or one complete dosing cycle is enough in case of switching due to a lack of response.

Patients with sustained skin clearance for at least 1 year, no recent flares and no active comorbidity, may be candidates for tapering of biological therapy. IL-23 inhibitors have demonstrated the most prolonged maintenance of psoriasis remission following treatment cessation among all biologic classes. This makes IL-23 inhibitors particularly suitable for situations where a planned drug-free period is necessary, such as surgery, pregnancy, or temporary contraindications. However, complete withdrawal is not recommended in any biologic class due to relapses.

Current guidelines provide only limited direction on dose adjustment, interval optimization or biologic holidays. Many decisions must rely on clinician experience or lower-level evidence. There is a pressing need for more high-quality data to guide these nuanced aspects of care. Future randomized trials and large-scale real-world studies are essential to establish evidence-based protocols for the flexible use of biologics. Such research will help refine treatment guidelines and empower dermatologists to make informed, individualized decisions, ultimately improving long-term outcomes, safety, and quality of life for patients with psoriasis.

Acknowledgements

All tables used in this chapter were prepared with Microsoft Word for formatting consistency.

Conflict of interest

The authors declare no conflict of interest and no funding source.

Author details

Muhammed Ali Mergen, Tubanur Çetinarslan and Aylin Türel Ermertcan*
Department of Dermatology and Venereology, Medical Faculty, Manisa Celal Bayar University, Manisa, Turkey

*Address all correspondence to: draylinturel@hotmail.com

References

[1] Bu J, Ding R, Zhou L, Chen X, Shen E. Epidemiology of psoriasis and comorbid diseases: A narrative review. Frontiers in Immunology. 2022;**13**:880201

[2] Parisi R, Symmons DP, Griffiths CE, Ashcroft DM. Identification and Management of Psoriasis and Associated ComorbidiTy (IMPACT) project team. Global epidemiology of psoriasis: A systematic review of incidence and prevalence. The Journal of Investigative Dermatology. 2013;**133**(2):377-385

[3] Tollefson MM, Crowson CS, McEvoy MT, Maradit Kremers H. Incidence of psoriasis in children: A population-based study. Journal of the American Academy of Dermatology. 2010;**62**(6):979-987

[4] Takeshita J, Grewal S, Langan SM, Mehta NN, Ogdie A, Van Voorhees AS, et al. Psoriasis and comorbid diseases: Epidemiology. Journal of the American Academy of Dermatology. 2017;**76**(3):377-390

[5] Nast A, Spuls PI, Dressler C, Bata-Csörgő Z, Bogdanov I, Boonen H, et al. EuroGuiDerm Guideline for the Systemic Treatment of Psoriasis Vulgaris. European Centre for Guidelines Development, European Dermatology Forum. Chareite dEBM. Sep 2023, partial update 2025

[6] Au SC, Madani A, Alhaddad M, Alkofide M, Gottlieb AB. Comparison of the efficacy of biologics versus conventional systemic therapies in the treatment of psoriasis at a comprehensive psoriasis care center. Journal of Drugs in Dermatology. 2013;**12**(8):861-866

[7] Garber C, Plotnikova N, Au SC, Sorensen EP, Gottlieb A. Biologic and conventional systemic therapies show similar safety and efficacy in elderly and adult patients with moderate to severe psoriasis. Journal of Drugs in Dermatology. 2015;**14**(8):846-852

[8] Menter A, Strober BE, Kaplan DH, Kivelevitch D, Prater EF, Stoff B, et al. Joint AAD-NPF guidelines of care for the management and treatment of psoriasis with biologics. Journal of the American Academy of Dermatology. 2019;**80**(4):1029-1072

[9] Feldman SR, Zhao Y, Shi L, Tran MH, Lu J. Economic and comorbidity burden among moderate-to-severe psoriasis patients with comorbid psoriatic arthritis. Arthritis Care & Research (Hoboken). 2015;**67**:708-717

[10] Amin M, Lee EB, Tsai TF, Wu JJ. Psoriasis and Co-morbidity. Acta Dermato-Venereologica. 2020;**100**(3):adv00033

[11] Raychaudhuri SP, Wilken R, Sukhov AC, Raychaudhuri SK, Maverakis E. Management of psoriatic arthritis: Early diagnosis, monitoring of disease severity and cutting edge therapies. Journal of Autoimmunity. 2017;**76**:21-37

[12] Cohen JM, Husni ME, Qureshi AA, Merola JF. Psoriatic arthritis: It's as easy as "PSA". Journal of the American Academy of Dermatology. 2015;**72**:905-906

[13] Pariser D, Schenkel B, Carter C, Farahi K, Brown TM, Ellis CN, et al. A multicenter, noninterventional study to evaluate patient–reported experiences of living with psoriasis. The Journal of Dermatological Treatment. 2016;**27**:19-26

[14] Edson-Heredia E, Zhu B, Guo J, Maeda-Chubachi T, Lebwohl M. Disease

burden and quality of life in psoriasis patients with and without comorbid psoriatic arthritis: Results from National Psoriasis Foundation panel surveys. Cutis. 2015;**95**:173-178

[15] Tillett W, Shaddick G, Askari A, Cooper A, Creamer P, Clunie G, et al. Factors influencing work disability in psoriatic arthritis: First results from a large UK multicentre study. Rheumatology. 2015;**54**:157-162

[16] Rahman P, Puig L, Gottlieb AB, Kavanaugh A, McInnes IB, Ritchlin C, et al. Ustekinumab treatment and improvement of physical function and health-related quality of life in patients with psoriatic arthritis. Arthritis Care and Research. 2016;**68**:1812-1822

[17] Amin M, No DJ, Egeberg A, Wu JJ. Choosing first-line biologic treatment for moderate-to-severe psoriasis: What does the evidence say? American Journal of Clinical Dermatology. 2018;**19**:1-3

[18] Fernández-Armenteros JM, Gómez-Arbonés X, Buti-Soler M, Betriu-Bars A, Sanmartin-Novell V, Ortega-Bravo M, et al. Psoriasis, metabolic syndrome and cardiovascular risk factors. A population-based study. Journal of the European Academy of Dermatology and Venereology. 2018;**33**:128-135

[19] Joshi AA, Lerman JB, Dey AK, Sajja AP, Belur AD, Elnabawi YA, et al. Association between aortic vascular inflammation and coronary artery plaque characteristics in psoriasis. JAMA Cardiology. 2018;**3**:949-956

[20] Dey AK, Joshi AA, Chaturvedi A, Lerman JB, Aberra TM, Rodante JA, et al. Association between skin and aortic vascular inflammation in patients with psoriasis: A case-cohort study using positron emission tomography/computed tomography. JAMA Cardiology. 2017;**2**:1013-1018

[21] Egeberg A, Skov L, Joshi AA, Mallbris L, Gislason GH, Wu JJ, et al. The relationship between duration of psoriasis, vascular inflammation, and cardiovascular events. Journal of the American Academy of Dermatology. 2017;**77**:650-656

[22] Wu JJ, Rowan CG, Bebchuk JD, Anthony MS. Association between tumor necrosis factor inhibitor (TNFi) therapy and changes in C-reactive protein (CRP), blood pressure, and alanine aminotransferase (ALT) among patients with psoriasis, psoriatic arthritis, or rheumatoid arthritis. Journal of the American Academy of Dermatology. 2015;**72**:917-919

[23] Wu JJ, Joshi AA, Reddy SP, Batech M, Egeberg A, Ahlehoff O, et al. Anti-inflammatory therapy with tumour necrosis factor inhibitors is associated with reduced risk of major adverse cardiovascular events in psoriasis. Journal of the European Academy of Dermatology and Venereology. 2018;**32**:1320-1326

[24] Wu JJ, Guérin A, Sundaram M, Dea K, Cloutier M, Mulani P. Cardiovascular event risk assessment in psoriasis patients treated with tumor necrosis factor-α inhibitors versus methotrexate. Journal of the American Academy of Dermatology. 2017;**76**:81-90

[25] Wu JJ, Sundaram M, Cloutier M, Gauthier-Loiselle M, Guérin A, Singh R, et al. The risk of cardiovascular events in psoriasis patients treated with tumor necrosis factor–α inhibitors versus phototherapy: An observational cohort study. Journal of the American Academy of Dermatology. 2018;**79**:60-68

[26] Hjuler KF, Bøttcher M, Vestergaard C, Bøtker HE, Iversen L, Kragballe K. Association between changes in coronary artery disease

progression and treatment with biologic agents for severe psoriasis. JAMA Dermatology. 2016;**152**:1114-1121

[27] Bissonnette R, Harel F, Krueger JG, Guertin MC, Chabot-Blanchet M, Gonzalez J, et al. TNF-α antagonist and vascular inflammation in patients with psoriasis vulgaris: A randomized placebo-controlled study. The Journal of Investigative Dermatology. 2017;**137**:1638-1645

[28] Mehta NN, Shin DB, Joshi AA, Dey AK, Armstrong AW, Duffin KC, et al. Effect of 2 psoriasis treatments on vascular inflammation and novel inflammatory cardiovascular biomarkers: A randomized placebo-controlled trial. Circulation. Cardiovascular Imaging. 2018;**11**:e007394

[29] Kumar S, Han J, Li T, et al. Obesity, waist circumference, weight change and the risk of psoriasis in US women. Journal of the European Academy of Dermatology and Venereology. 2013;**27**(10):1293-1298

[30] Armstrong AW, Harskamp CT, Armstrong EJ. The association between psoriasis and obesity: A systematic review and meta-analysis of observational studies. Nutrition & Diabetes. 2012;**2**:e54

[31] Armstrong AW, Harskamp CT, Armstrong EJ. Psoriasis and metabolic syndrome: A systematic review and meta-analysis of observational studies. Journal of the American Academy of Dermatology. 2013;**68**(4):654-662

[32] Langan SM, Seminara NM, Shin DB, et al. Prevalence of metabolic syndrome in patients with psoriasis: A population-based study in the United Kingdom. The Journal of Investigative Dermatology. 2012;**132**(3 Pt 1):556-562

[33] Cohen AD, Dreiher J, Birkenfeld S. Psoriasis associated with ulcerative colitis and Crohn's disease. Journal of the European Academy of Dermatology and Venereology. 2009;**23**(5):561-565

[34] Li WQ, Han JL, Chan AT, et al. Psoriasis, psoriatic arthritis and increased risk of incident Crohn's disease in U.S. women. Annals of the Rheumatic Diseases. 2013;**72**(7):1200-1205

[35] Wu JJ, Penfold RB, Primatesta P, Fox TK, Stewart C, Reddy SP, et al. The risk of depression, suicidal ideation and suicide attempt in patients with psoriasis, psoriatic arthritis or ankylosing spondylitis. Journal of the European Academy of Dermatology and Venereology. 2017;**31**:1168-1175

[36] Lewinson RT, Vallerand IA, Lowerison MW, Parsons LM, Frolkis AD, Kaplan GG, et al. Depression is associated with an increased risk of psoriatic arthritis among patients with psoriasis: A population-based study. The Journal of Investigative Dermatology. 2017;**137**:828-835

[37] Egeberg A, Khalid U, Hilmar Gislason G, Mallbris L, Skov L, Riis HP. Impact of depression on risk of myocardial infarction, stroke and cardiovascular death in patients with psoriasis: A Danish Nationwide study. Acta Dermato-Venereologica. 2016;**96**:218-222

[38] Aberra TM, Joshi AA, Lerman JB, Rodante JA, Dahiya AK, Teague HL, et al. Self-reported depression in psoriasis is associated with subclinical vascular diseases. Atherosclerosis. 2016;**251**:219-225

[39] Wu JJ, Feldman SR, Koo J, Marangell LB. Epidemiology of mental health comorbidity in psoriasis. The Journal of Dermatological Treatment. 2018;**29**:487-495

[40] Oliveira Mde F, Rocha Bde O, Duarte GV. Psoriasis: Classical and emerging comorbidities. Anais Brasileiros de Dermatologia. 2015;**90**:9-20

[41] Wang Y, Chen Y, Yu Q, Shi Y. Biologic and small-molecule therapies for moderate-to-severe psoriasis: Focus on psoriasis comorbidities. BioDrugs. 2023;**37**(1):35-55

[42] Langley RG, Krueger GG, Griffiths CE. Psoriasis: Epidemiology, clinical features, and quality of life. Annals of the Rheumatic Diseases. 2005;**64 Suppl 2**(Suppl. 2):ii18-ii23; discussion ii24-5

[43] Gisondi P, Talamonti M, Chiricozzi A, Piaserico S, Amerio P, Balato A, et al. Treat-to-target approach for the management of patients with moderate-to-severe plaque psoriasis: Consensus recommendations. Dermatology and Therapy. 2021;**11**(1):235-252

[44] Mrowietz U, Kragballe K, Reich K, Spuls P, Griffiths CE, Nast A, et al. Definition of treatment goals for moderate to severe psoriasis: A European consensus. Archives of Dermatological Research. 2011;**303**(1):1-10

[45] Smith CH, Yiu ZZN, Bale T, Burden AD, Coates LC, Edwards W, et al. British Association of Dermatologists guidelines for biologic therapy for psoriasis 2020: A rapid update. British Journal of Dermatology. 2020;**183**(4):628-637

[46] Gordon KB, Foley P, Krueger JG, Pinter A, Reich K, Vender R, et al. Bimekizumab efficacy and safety in moderate to severe plaque psoriasis (BE READY): A multicentre, double-blind, placebo-controlled, randomised withdrawal phase 3 trial. Lancet. 2021;**397**(10273):475-486

[47] Wang TS, Tsai TF. Biologics switch in psoriasis. Immunotherapy. 2019;**11**(6):531-541

[48] Augustin M, Reich K, Yamauchi P, Pinter A, Bagel J, Dahale S, et al. Secukinumab dosing every 2 weeks demonstrated superior efficacy compared with dosing every 4 weeks in patients with psoriasis weighing 90 kg or more: Results of a randomized controlled trial. The British Journal of Dermatology. 2022;**186**(6):942-954

[49] Wu JJ, Patel M, Zeng F, Huang A, Pan X, Cao Y, et al. Real-world dose escalation of biologics for moderate-to-severe psoriasis in the United States. The Journal of Dermatological Treatment. 2023;**34**(1):2200869

[50] Mufti A, Maliyar K, Walton L, Vender R, Yeung J. Guselkumab dosing interval optimization in adult patients with psoriasis: A retrospective, multicenter case series. Journal of the American Academy of Dermatology. 2020;**83**(6):1813-1814

[51] Bagel J, Novak K, Nelson E. Adjunctive use of halobetasol propionate-tazarotene in biologic-experienced patients with psoriasis. Cutis. 2022;**109**(2):103-109

[52] Jensen JD, Delcambre MR, Nguyen G, Sami N. Biologic therapy with or without topical treatment in psoriasis: What does the current evidence say? American Journal of Clinical Dermatology. 2014;**15**(5):379-385

[53] Hou YL, Lin SH. Real-world efficacy of adjunctive calcipotriene/betamethasone dipropionate foam for recalcitrant psoriatic lesions on the scalp or lower legs with biologic therapy. The Journal of Dermatology. 2023;**50**(10):1272-1278

[54] Bagel J, Nelson E, Zapata J, Hetzel A. Adjunctive use of calcipotriene/ betamethasone dipropionate foam in a real-world setting curtails the cost of biologics without reducing efficacy in psoriasis. Dermatology and Therapy. 2020;**10**(6):1383-1396

[55] Zachariae C, Mork NJ, Reunala T, et al. The combination of etanercept and methotrexate increases the effectiveness of treatment in active psoriasis despite inadequate effect of methotrexate therapy. Acta Dermato-Venereologica. 2008;**88**:495-501

[56] Gisondi P, Del Giglio M, Cotena C, Girolomoni G. Combining etanercept and acitretin in the therapy of chronic plaque psoriasis: A 24-week, randomized, controlled, investigator-blinded pilot trial. The British Journal of Dermatology. 2008;**158**:1345-1349

[57] Smith CH, Anstey AV, Barker JN, et al. British Association of Dermatologists' guidelines for biologic interventions for psoriasis 2009. The British Journal of Dermatology. 2009;**161**:987-1019

[58] Nakamura M, Koo J. Safety considerations with combination therapies for psoriasis. Expert Opinion on Drug Safety. 2020;**19**(4):489-498

[59] Bonomo L, Abittan BJ, Hashim PW, Karki C, Mason M, Lebwohl M. Combination use of systemic therapies in psoriasis: Baseline characteristics from the corrona psoriasis registry. Journal of Drugs in Dermatology. 2019;**18**(8):731-740

[60] Jeong YD, Jo H, Cho H, Jang W, Park J, Lee S, et al. Biologics use for psoriasis during pregnancy and its related adverse outcomes in pregnant women and newborns: Findings from WHO pharmacovigilance study. International Archives of Allergy and Immunology. 2025;**186**(6):579-593

[61] Mrowietz U, de Jong EM, Kragballe K, Langley R, Nast A, Puig L, et al. A consensus report on appropriate treatment optimization and transitioning in the management of moderate-to-severe plaque psoriasis. Journal of the European Academy of Dermatology and Venereology. 2014;**28**(4):438-453

[62] Armstrong AW, Patel M, Li C, Garg V, Mandava MR, Wu JJ. Real-world switching patterns and associated characteristics in patients with psoriasis treated with biologics in the United States. The Journal of Dermatological Treatment. 2023;**34**(1):2200870

[63] Tsai YC, Tsai TF. Switching biologics in psoriasis—Practical guidance and evidence to support. Expert Review of Clinical Pharmacology. 2020;**13**(5):493-503

[64] Megna M, Fabbrocini G, Ruggiero A, Cinelli E. Efficacy and safety of risankizumab in psoriasis patients who failed anti-IL-17, anti-12/23 and/or anti IL-23: Preliminary data of a real-life 16-week retrospective study. Dermatologic Therapy. 2020;**33**(6):e14144

[65] Williams VL, Cohen PR. TNF alpha antagonist-induced lupus-like syndrome: Report and review of the literature with implications for treatment with alternative TNF alpha antagonists. International Journal of Dermatology. 2011;**50**(5):619-625

[66] Wehrmann C, Sondermann W, Körber A. Secukinumab-induced subacute-cutaneous lupus erythematosus. Der Hautarzt. 2018;**69**(1):64-66

[67] Jeong YD, Jo H, Cho H, Jang W, Park J, Lee S, et al. Biologics use for psoriasis during pregnancy and its related adverse outcomes in pregnant women and newborns: Findings from WHO pharmacovigilance study. International Archives of Allergy and Immunology. 2024:1-15

[68] Atalay S, van den Reek JMPA, van Vugt LJ, Otero ME, van de Kerkhof PCM, den Broeder AA, et al. Tight controlled dose reduction of biologics in psoriasis patients with low disease activity: A randomized pragmatic non-inferiority trial. BMC Dermatology. 2017;**17**(1):6

[69] Atalay S, van den Reek JMPA, den Broeder AA, van Vugt LJ, Otero ME, Njoo MD, et al. Comparison of tightly controlled dose reduction of biologics with usual care for patients with psoriasis: A randomized clinical trial. JAMA Dermatology. 2020;**156**(4):393-400

[70] Brezinski EA, Armstrong AW. Off-label biologic regimens in psoriasis: A systematic review of efficacy and safety of dose escalation, reduction, and interrupted biologic therapy. PLoS ONE. 2012;**7**(4):e33486

[71] Masson Regnault M, Shourick J, Jendoubi F, et al. Time to relapse after discontinuing systemic treatment for psoriasis: A systematic review. American Journal of Clinical Dermatology. 2022;**23**:433-447

[72] Hsieh CY, Hsu FL, Tsai TF. Comparison of drug-free remission after the end of phase III trials of three different anti-IL-23 inhibitors in psoriasis. Dermatology and Therapy. 2024;**14**(9):2607-2620

[73] Chiu HY, Hui RC, Tsai TF, Chen YC, Chang Liao NF, Chen PH, et al. Predictors of time to relapse following ustekinumab withdrawal in patients with psoriasis who had responded to therapy: An 8-year multicenter study. Journal of the American Academy of Dermatology. 2023;**88**(1):71-78

[74] Papp KA, Langley RG, Lebwohl M, Krueger GG, Szapary P, et al. Efficacy and safety of ustekinumab, a human interleukin-12/23 monoclonal antibody, in patients with psoriasis: 52-week results from a randomised, double-blind, placebo-controlled trial (PHOENIX 2). Lancet. 2008;**371**:1675-1684

[75] Leonardi CL, Kimball AB, Papp KA, Yeilding N, Guzzo C, et al. Efficacy and safety of ustekinumab, a human interleukin-12/23 monoclonal antibody, in patients with psoriasis: 76-week results from a randomised, double-blind, placebo-controlled trial (PHOENIX 1). Lancet. 2008;**371**:1665-1674

[76] Mrowietz U, Leonardi CL, Girolomoni G, Toth D, Morita A, Balki SA, et al. Secukinumab retreatment-as-needed versus fixed-interval maintenance regimen for moderate to severe plaque psoriasis: A randomized, double-blind, noninferiority trial (SCULPTURE). Journal of the American Academy of Dermatology. 2015;**73**(1):27-36.e1

[77] Coates LC, Pillai SG, Tahir H, Valter I, Chandran V, Kameda H, et al. Withdrawing ixekizumab in patients with psoriatic arthritis who achieved minimal disease activity: Results from a randomized, double-blind withdrawal study. Arthritis & Rhematology. 2021;**73**(9):1663-1672

[78] Eyerich K, Asadullah K, Pinter A, Weisenseel P, Reich K, Paul C, et al. Noninferiority of 16-week vs 8-week guselkumab dosing in super responders for maintaining control of psoriasis: The GUIDE randomized clinical trial. JAMA

Dermatology. 2024;**160**(9):953-963. DOI: 10.1001/jamadermatol.2024.2463. Erratum in: JAMA Dermatology 2024; 160(11):1257

[79] Krueger GG, Papp KA, Stough DB, Loven KH, Gulliver WP, et al. A randomized, double-blind, placebo-controlled phase III study evaluating efficacy and tolerability of 2 courses of alefacept in patients with chronic plaque psoriasis. Journal of the American Academy of Dermatology. 2002;**47**:821-833

[80] Kirby B, Chiricozzi A, Gorecki P, Buyze J, Parker R, Wegner S, et al. Time to loss of disease control following guselkumab withdrawal in relation to initial speed of response: A post hoc analysis of the VOYAGE 2 trial. Dermatology. 2024;**241**(2):133-142

[81] Tian D, Lai Y. The relapse of psoriasis: Mechanisms and mysteries. JID Innovations. 2022;**2**(3):100116

[82] Norden A, Moon JY, Javadi SS, Munawar L, Maul JT, Wu JJ. Anti-drug antibodies of IL-23 inhibitors for psoriasis: A systematic review. Journal of the European Academy of Dermatology and Venereology. 2022;**36**(8):1171-1177

[83] Gordon KB, Armstrong AW, Foley P, Song M, Shen YK, Li S, et al. Guselkumab efficacy after withdrawal is associated with suppression of serum IL-23-regulated IL-17 and IL-22 in psoriasis: VOYAGE 2 study. The Journal of Investigative Dermatology. 2019;**139**(12):2437-2446.e1

Chapter 3

Practical Management of Psoriasis in Special Clinical Circumstances

Selda Pelin Kartal and Tuğcan Yüksek

Abstract

This chapter thoroughly discusses the management strategies for psoriasis within complex clinical scenarios and special patient groups. It examines therapeutic options and safety considerations for systemic and biologic therapies in patients who have coexisting hepatic or renal disease, cardiovascular issues, malignancies, or inflammatory bowel disease, and addresses specific cases such as pregnancy and lactation. Furthermore, the management of psoriasis complicated by psoriatic arthritis, latent tuberculosis, or neurological disorders such as multiple sclerosis is detailed. The chapter emphasizes evidence-based, personalized treatment approaches informed by contemporary clinical trials and real-life patient data.

Keywords: psoriasis, treatment algorithm, pregnancy, malignancy, psoriatic arthritis, biologic therapy, guideline

1. Introduction

Psoriasis is a chronic inflammatory skin condition linked with significant systemic complications and numerous comorbidities. Although standard treatments often effectively control disease activity in many patients, certain clinical circumstances, including pregnancy, impaired organ function, cancer, and coexisting autoimmune or infectious disorders, require customized therapeutic approaches. Managing psoriasis in these specific groups involves carefully balancing treatment efficacy with safety, taking into account altered drug metabolism, immune-related risks, and particular vulnerabilities. This chapter provides a practical, evidence-based framework to support clinical decision-making in complex psoriasis cases, focusing on achieving optimal dermatological outcomes and integrated multidisciplinary care.

2. Pregnancy and breastfeeding

The effect of pregnancy on psoriasis is variable; symptoms may improve in some patients yet worsen in others, highlighting the need for individualized therapeutic strategies based on clinical presentation and established safety profiles. Topical therapies remain the cornerstone of treatment for mild psoriasis during pregnancy. Emollients and oatmeal-based baths are universally safe and should be used liberally to maintain skin barrier function and reduce inflammation. Low- to moderate-potency topical corticosteroids are preferred, particularly when applied in limited quantities to localized plaques. High-potency corticosteroids may be used cautiously for short periods in refractory cases but are associated with potential risks, including fetal growth restriction if extensively applied or used long-term. Topical calcineurin inhibitors, such as tacrolimus and pimecrolimus, although off-label in pregnancy, are considered relatively safe for sensitive areas such as the face and intertriginous zones due to their minimal systemic absorption [1].

Phototherapy, specifically NB-UVB, is considered safe for treating moderate-to-severe psoriasis throughout all trimesters and poses no known risk to the fetus; however, as prolonged NB-UVB therapy may lower maternal folate levels, supplementing with folic acid during early pregnancy is recommended. While a standard course of NB-UVB treatment did not affect serum or red blood cell folate levels in psoriasis patients, El-Saie et al. found that high cumulative doses of NB-UVB led to folate photodegradation and a reduction in serum folate levels, with this effect being directly linked to the total cumulative dose, highlighting the potential risk associated with prolonged NB-UVB therapy [2, 3]. In contrast, psoralen plus ultraviolet A (PUVA) therapy is contraindicated during pregnancy due to its mutagenic potential and should be avoided entirely [4].

In patients requiring systemic treatment, cyclosporine remains the most studied and accepted systemic agent during pregnancy. Short-term use at the lowest effective dose is recommended, and careful monitoring for hypertension and nephrotoxicity is essential. Among biologic therapies, TNF-α inhibitors are the preferred class for use during pregnancy [5]. Certolizumab pegol, in particular, is favored due to its lack of an Fc fragment, which minimizes placental transfer. The CRIB study confirmed negligible fetal exposure to certolizumab pegol, establishing it as the biologic of choice for pregnant women requiring systemic disease control [6]. Etanercept, a fusion protein, exhibits substantially lower placental transfer than IgG1 monoclonal antibodies such as adalimumab and infliximab, with reported cord blood:maternal serum ratios as low as 1:14 [7]. Importantly, the use of TNF inhibitor exposure after the 20th gestational week should be minimized as they have been associated with persistence of the drug in neonatal serum for several months, prompting recommendations to avoid live vaccines, such as BCG, for at least 6 months postpartum. On the other hand, current data have not demonstrated any increased risk of congenital malformations or low birth weight associated with in utero exposure to TNF-α inhibitors [5].

Data on IL-17 and IL-23 inhibitors during pregnancy are limited, and these agents should generally be avoided unless no safer alternative exists and disease severity mandates their use [5]. Agents that are unequivocally contraindicated during pregnancy include methotrexate, acitretin, and topical retinoids such as tazarotene. Methotrexate is highly teratogenic and associated with pregnancy loss and congenital anomalies including microcephaly, craniosynostosis, tetralogy of Fallot and limb defects [8]. Acitretin possesses a notably prolonged elimination half-life, significantly increasing the risk of severe teratogenic effects; consequently, reliable contraception must be maintained for an extended duration even following cessation of therapy. Similarly, topical tazarotene, classified as a retinoid derivative, is contraindicated during pregnancy due to its recognized teratogenic potential [9].

Most topical therapies, including emollients and low-potency corticosteroids, are considered safe during lactation, provided that medications are not directly applied to the nipple-areola complex prior to nursing. NB-UVB phototherapy remains a safe option. Certolizumab pegol is again the preferred biologic during breastfeeding due to its minimal secretion into breast milk. Other TNF-α inhibitors may also be acceptable but require case-by-case evaluation, ideally in consultation with pediatrics. Methotrexate, acitretin, and tazarotene are contraindicated during breastfeeding because of potential drug transfer and toxic effects on the infant [10].

3. Hepatic impairment

The management of psoriasis in patients with hepatic impairment requires particular caution due to the hepatic metabolism of many systemic therapies and the frequent co-occurrence of liver disease, especially non-alcoholic fatty liver disease (NAFLD). Psoriasis patients have up to a twofold increased risk of NAFLD, driven by shared risk factors such as metabolic syndrome, obesity, and chronic inflammation. Careful selection of therapy is essential to avoid further hepatic injury while achieving disease control [11].

Baseline evaluation should include liver function tests (ALT, AST, GGT, ALP, bilirubin) and mandatory screening for hepatitis B and C (HBsAg, anti-HBc, anti-HBs). Imaging studies, including liver ultrasound or transient elastography, may be necessary to assess fibrosis. In patients with cirrhosis or decompensated liver disease, systemic immunosuppressives should be used with extreme caution or avoided altogether [12].

For mild cases, treatment primarily involves topical therapies such as emollients, corticosteroids of low to moderate potency, vitamin D analogs, and calcineurin inhibitors. Additionally, NB-UVB phototherapy serves as a highly effective, non-hepatotoxic alternative for patients with extensive disease who are unsuitable for systemic treatment [13].

Methotrexate, a key systemic therapy for moderate-to-severe psoriasis, carries a notable risk of liver toxicity. It can lead to cumulative liver fibrosis and, in rare instances, cirrhosis. Patients with any pre-existing liver issues should generally avoid methotrexate. Additionally, non-invasive tests like FibroScan or a liver biopsy might be necessary when considering long-term methotrexate treatment. Similarly, acitretin, although primarily metabolized hepatically, is associated with alterations in lipid metabolism and potential hepatotoxicity, making it an unfavorable option in patients with active liver disease or dyslipidemia [14].

Cyclosporine, another systemic agent with hepatic metabolism, may cause cholestasis or hepatocellular injury, though less commonly than nephrotoxicity. Its use should be reserved for short-term indications in carefully monitored patients with only mild hepatic impairment, and it should be avoided in cases of significant liver dysfunction. On the other hand, the oral phosphodiesterase-4 inhibitor apremilast is generally well-tolerated in patients with hepatic impairment and does not require dose adjustment in mild to moderate liver dysfunction [14].

Biologic therapies offer a safer alternative for psoriatic patients with hepatic comorbidities. IL-17 (secukinumab, ixekizumab) and IL-23 inhibitors (guselkumab, risankizumab, tildrakizumab) are metabolized primarily by proteolysis, avoiding hepatic cytochrome P450 pathways. Long-term data have not shown increased hepatotoxicity with these agents [15].

Ustekinumab, an IL-12/23 inhibitor, has been used successfully in hepatitis B carriers; however, cohort data report a 17.4% reactivation rate in HBsAg-positive patients not receiving antiviral prophylaxis, while no reactivations occurred in those on prophylaxis [16]. Similarly, TNF-α inhibitors carry a substantial risk of hepatitis B virus (HBV) reactivation, particularly with infliximab and adalimumab. Reactivation rates up to 39% have been reported in HBsAg-positive patients without prophylaxis, compared to less than 10% in those receiving antiviral therapy [17].

IL-17 inhibitors appear safer in this context. A prospective study reported 0% reactivation in patients receiving secukinumab alongside antiviral prophylaxis, versus 15.2% without it. While IL-23 inhibitors have limited data, no HBV reactivation has been reported in phase III trials, though rare isolated cases exist. Their safety profile remains promising for HBsAg-negative/anti-HBc-positive patients and may be cautiously considered under antiviral cover [15, 18].

For patients with chronic hepatitis B infection, antiviral prophylaxis with nucleoside analogs should be initiated before starting immunosuppressive therapy to reduce the risk of reactivation. Prophylaxis should continue for 6 to 12 months after treatment cessation, particularly for TNF-α and IL-12/23 blockers. For patients with hepatitis C infection, recent advances in antiviral therapy have improved the management of coexistent HCV and psoriasis, allowing more flexibility in systemic treatment selection once viral eradication is achieved [15].

Ultimately, management of psoriasis in the setting of hepatic impairment requires an individualized approach. Topical and phototherapeutic options should be optimized, hepatotoxic systemic agents minimized, and biologic therapies should be selected preferentially where indicated. Close collaboration with hepatologists is advisable for complex cases involving advanced fibrosis, cirrhosis, or concomitant viral hepatitis.

4. Renal impairment

Renal impairment presents a significant clinical challenge in the management of psoriasis, given the altered pharmacokinetics of many systemic therapies and the increased susceptibility to drug-induced nephrotoxicity. Chronic kidney disease (CKD) is more prevalent among patients with moderate-to-severe psoriasis compared to the general population, with systemic inflammation, hypertension, diabetes, and medication side effects contributing to renal decline. Furthermore, psoriasis itself has been recognized as a systemic inflammatory condition capable of promoting endothelial dysfunction and renal injury independently of traditional risk factors [13].

Comprehensive baseline renal evaluation is mandatory before initiating systemic treatment in psoriatic patients, particularly those with known risk factors or comorbidities. Laboratory assessments should include serum creatinine, estimated glomerular filtration rate (eGFR), blood urea nitrogen (BUN), electrolytes, and urinalysis to detect proteinuria or hematuria. In patients with moderate (eGFR 30–59 mL/min/1.73 m^2) or severe (eGFR <30) renal impairment, systemic therapy selection must be adjusted accordingly to minimize further renal insult [19].

For patients with limited cutaneous involvement, topical therapies remain the primary treatment option and pose no risk to renal function. Emollients, corticosteroids, vitamin D analogs, and topical calcineurin inhibitors are all safe. Narrowband UVB phototherapy also provides an effective and kidney-friendly treatment modality, particularly valuable in patients with moderate-to-severe disease who are not candidates for systemic immunomodulation. In cases requiring systemic intervention, biologics and certain oral agents offer safer profiles compared to traditional immunosuppressants. **Table 1** summarizes the renal safety, dialysis compatibility, and known adverse events of systemic psoriasis treatments.

Systemic agent	Use in CKD	Use in dialysis	Renal adverse events
Methotrexate	Contraindicated in eGFR <60	Not recommended	Risk of toxic accumulation, myelosuppression, mucositis
Cyclosporine	Avoid due to dose-dependent nephrotoxicity	Not recommended	Acute and chronic nephrotoxicity, hypertension
Acitretin	Use with caution	Caution advised	No direct renal toxicity; worsen hyperlipidemia, xerosis
Apremilast	Safe with dose reduction if eGFR <30	Can be used at 30 mg/day	Rare case reports of renal tubular acidosis
TNF-α inhibitors	Safe in stable renal function	Can be used; off-dialysis day	Rare acute kidney injury; infection risk in CKD
IL-17 inhibitors	Safe; no renal clearance required	Can be used; off-dialysis day	No reported renal adverse events
IL-23 inhibitors	Safe; primarily cleared proteolytically	Can be used; off-dialysis day	No reported renal adverse events
Ustekinumab	Safe; no dose adjustment needed	Can be used; off-dialysis day	No renal toxicity observed in trials or registries

Table 1.
Renal safety and dialysis considerations of systemic treatments for psoriasis [9, 19–21].

5. Diabetes mellitus

Patients with moderate-to-severe psoriasis are at significantly increased risk for developing type 2 diabetes, independent of obesity or metabolic syndrome. This is largely driven by chronic systemic inflammation involving TNF-α, IL-6, and IL-17, which contribute to insulin resistance and endothelial dysfunction. A baseline workup should include HbA1c, lipid profile, blood pressure, BMI, and screening for diabetic complications, such as nephropathy and retinopathy, which may impact treatment selection [22].

Topical therapies and NB-UVB phototherapy remain safe options for limited or moderate disease, with no adverse effects on glycemic control. Prolonged use of potent topical corticosteroids should be limited due to potential systemic absorption and glucose dysregulation [23].

Among systemic agents, methotrexate requires close hepatic monitoring because diabetics are at higher risk for NAFLD. Acitretin can exacerbate dyslipidemia and should be avoided in patients with poorly controlled lipid profiles or cardiovascular disease. Cyclosporine is usually not favored due to potential side effects like hypertension, nephrotoxicity, and increased insulin resistance; its link to new-onset diabetes has been well-established in transplant patients [12].

Apremilast has shown a metabolically neutral profile and favorable safety in real-world use among diabetic patients. Observational studies indicate that it does not lead to insulin resistance and may promote modest weight loss, offering additional benefit in overweight individuals with psoriasis [24].

Biologic therapies are extensively utilized among diabetic patients and demonstrate excellent safety profiles. TNF-α inhibitors, such as adalimumab and etanercept, have shown modest improvements in insulin sensitivity in some cohorts [25]. IL-17 and IL-23 inhibitors are metabolically neutral and have not been associated with worsening glucose levels in real-world studies [26]. Moreover, by reducing systemic inflammation, these agents may indirectly contribute to improved metabolic homeostasis, particularly in patients with underlying insulin resistance or metabolic syndrome. Ustekinumab (anti-IL12/23) is similarly safe and convenient for patients managing multiple comorbidities due to its long dosing interval [12].

Close collaboration with endocrinology, careful monitoring of metabolic parameters, and patient education regarding lifestyle modification are essential components of successful long-term management.

6. Congestive heart failure

Congestive heart failure (CHF) is an important comorbidity that influences treatment decisions in patients with moderate-to-severe psoriasis. The presence of CHF complicates psoriasis management due to the cardiovascular risks associated with several systemic treatments, particularly biologic agents targeting the TNF-α pathway. Therefore, careful assessment of cardiac function and tailored therapeutic strategies are essential for safe and effective management [27].

Baseline evaluation of psoriatic patients with known or suspected CHF should include determination of the New York Heart Association (NYHA) functional class and measurement of left ventricular ejection fraction (LVEF). Patients with NYHA class III or IV symptoms or an LVEF less than 40% are considered high-risk and require especially cautious therapeutic selection [13].

In terms of conventional systemic therapies, methotrexate may be cautiously considered in patients with stable, compensated CHF. Although observational studies in psoriasis suggest methotrexate may reduce cardiovascular risk by lowering inflammation, a recent cohort study found no difference in ischemic heart disease rates between methotrexate and other nonbiologic treatments. Regardless, careful monitoring of fluid balance, renal function, and hematologic parameters is necessary during methotrexate therapy in CHF patients [28, 29]. Acitretin, while not directly cardiotoxic, may exacerbate hyperlipidemia, a known contributor to atherosclerotic progression and heart failure. Its use should be limited or avoided in patients with poorly controlled lipid profiles or established coronary artery disease [30]. Cyclosporine, owing to its effects on sodium and water retention, hypertension, and nephrotoxicity, is contraindicated in moderate-to-severe CHF. Use of cyclosporine in this patient population can precipitate or worsen CHF and is generally avoided [28].

Biologic therapies offer substantial efficacy in psoriasis, but their use must be carefully considered in the context of CHF. TNF-α inhibitors, such as infliximab and etanercept, have been associated with worsening heart failure, particularly at higher doses [31]. Randomized clinical trials in heart failure populations demonstrated increased mortality and hospitalization rates with TNF-α blockade in NYHA class III–IV patients [32]. Consequently, TNF inhibitors are contraindicated in patients with advanced CHF. Even in NYHA class I–II CHF, TNF-α inhibitors should only be considered after consultation with a cardiologist and a baseline echocardiography. Treatment should be discontinued if symptoms worsen or ejection fraction drops below 50% [33].

In contrast, IL-17 inhibitors and IL-23 inhibitors have demonstrated no increased risk of new-onset or worsening CHF in clinical trials or post-marketing registries. A pooled analysis of long-term ixekizumab trials involving 3736 patients reported no CHF exacerbations [34]. A meta-analysis also confirmed no significant risk of new-onset CHF with IL-17 or IL-23 inhibitors [35]. Their favorable cardiac safety profile,

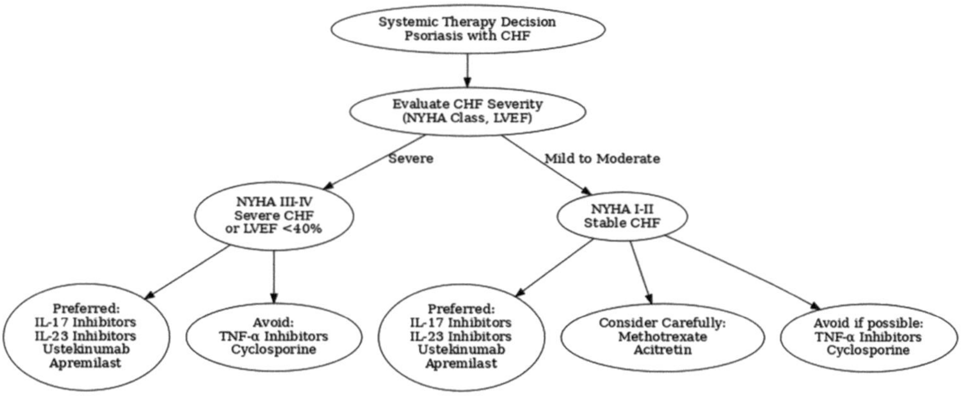

Figure 1.
Clinical treatment algorithm for psoriasis management in patients with congestive heart failure.

rapid onset of action, and strong efficacy in both skin and joint involvement make them well-suited for psoriatic patients with coexisting heart failure requiring systemic treatment. While long-term cardiovascular outcome data are more extensive for IL-17 inhibitors, available evidence for IL-23 inhibitors, including guselkumab and risankizumab, remains reassuring, with no signal of adverse cardiac events reported to date. Ustekinumab, likewise demonstrates a reassuring cardiac safety profile and may be an alternative choice, particularly for patients with concomitant arthritis or inflammatory bowel disease [36]. A summarized treatment algorithm outlining the clinical approach to psoriasis management in patients with CHF is presented in **Figure 1**.

7. Neurologic disorders

The association between psoriasis and neurologic disorders, particularly multiple sclerosis (MS), has garnered increasing attention due to overlapping immunopathogenic mechanisms and the potential impact of systemic therapies on neural tissues. Both psoriasis and MS are characterized by dysregulation of T-cell-mediated immune responses, notably involving the IL-17/Th17 axis [37]. Importantly, several treatments for psoriasis, especially TNF-α inhibitors, have been implicated in either exacerbating or inducing demyelinating disorders, necessitating cautious therapeutic planning in patients with neurologic comorbidities [19].

Prior to initiating systemic therapy in patients with psoriasis and a history of demyelinating disease, a comprehensive neurologic evaluation is essential. Patients with unexplained neurologic symptoms such as visual disturbances, muscle weakness, sensory changes, or gait abnormalities should be thoroughly investigated to rule out latent or subclinical MS. Similarly, a family history of MS or other autoimmune neurologic diseases should prompt heightened vigilance in systemic therapy selection [38].

When systemic therapy is required in psoriatic patients with comorbid neurological disorders, conventional agents such as methotrexate and acitretin are generally considered safe. Neither has been associated with central demyelination, although rare cases of reversible leukoencephalopathy and cognitive effects have been reported with low-dose methotrexate [39]. Cyclosporine is associated with neurotoxic side effects in up to 28% of patients, including tremor, paresthesia, seizures, and cognitive changes [40]. These effects are dose-dependent and more likely in settings of blood-brain barrier disruption. Given its narrow therapeutic window, nephrotoxicity, and potential for neurotoxicity, cyclosporine should be used cautiously and only when other agents are contraindicated. Apremilast is considered safe in demyelinating diseases, with no known CNS toxicity. It does not cross the blood-brain barrier and is particularly appealing in MS patients who suffer from limited mobility or metabolic comorbidities due to its weight-reducing effect and favorable safety profile [41].

TNF-α inhibitors are contraindicated in MS due to strong mechanistic and clinical evidence linking them to central and peripheral demyelination [42]. All five TNF inhibitors, including the newer agents certolizumab and golimumab, have been implicated in new-onset or worsening MS, with real-world reports showing most events occur within the first year of therapy [43]. Among 84 reported cases of psoriasis, only 33% achieved full recovery after stopping treatment, while several progressed or showed new silent lesions. Consequently, TNF-α inhibitors should be strictly avoided in this population [44].

IL-17 inhibitors, particularly secukinumab, are currently regarded as the most appropriate biologic class for patients with psoriasis and coexisting MS, given that IL-17A and IL-17F levels have been implicated in the pathogenesis of both conditions. Clinical trial data involving patients with relapsing-remitting MS revealed a 49% reduction in new MRI lesions and a 67% reduction in active lesions with secukinumab treatment [45]. Real-world evidence further supports its safety: in a small series, 80% of patients with both MS and psoriasis who were treated with secukinumab remained clinically stable, with no progression of neurologic disease and no reported cases of de novo central demyelination [44]. For other IL-17 inhibitors, such as ixekizumab and bimekizumab, no robust data are currently available. To date, only a single case report suggests the safe use of ixekizumab in a patient with pre-existing multiple sclerosis, and there are no published neurologic safety data for bimekizumab [46].

Ustekinumab, targeting both IL-12 and IL-23, is another biologic agent with a reassuring neurologic safety profile [47]. IL-23 inhibitors, including guselkumab, risankizumab, and tildrakizumab, are also regarded as safe choices in this setting. Although long-term neurologic outcome data are still emerging, there is currently no evidence suggesting that IL-23 blockade promotes demyelination [48, 49].

8. Latent tuberculosis and HIV

Management of psoriasis in patients with latent tuberculosis (TB) requires careful screening and strategic treatment selection, especially prior to the initiation of systemic immunosuppressive agents. Interferon-gamma release assays (IGRAs) such as QuantiFERON-TB Gold are preferred over tuberculin skin tests (TST) in BCG-vaccinated individuals. A chest X-ray is essential to rule out active TB. If latent TB is confirmed, chemoprophylaxis, typically with isoniazid for 6–9 months, should be started. Most guidelines allow systemic therapy to begin after 1 month of prophylaxis, though this may vary by region. Close clinical and radiological monitoring throughout treatment is strongly advised [50].

Among systemic agents, TNF-α inhibitors pose the highest risk of TB reactivation. TNF is essential for granuloma integrity and host control of *Mycobacterium tuberculosis*. Conventional systemic therapies, including methotrexate and cyclosporine, have lower TB reactivation potential, but screening and vigilance are still required. TB reactivation with these agents is rare but reported, particularly in long-term use or when combined with other immunosuppressants [51].

Apremilast and acitretin, given their non-immunosuppressive mechanism of action, have not been associated with TB reactivation. They do not require prophylaxis and are safe options for psoriasis patients with LTBI, particularly those ineligible for biologic therapies [17, 21].

Ustekinumab has shown a low risk of TB reactivation in clinical trials (0/3177 cases with prophylaxis); however, recent pharmacovigilance data from the FAERS database reported 121 cases of latent TB, indicating a potential real-world signal and reinforcing the need for strict pre-treatment screening and ongoing monitoring [52, 53].

IL-17 and IL-23 inhibitors have shown an excellent safety profile regarding tuberculosis reactivation, with no reported cases in large clinical trials involving 3430 patients treated with secukinumab, 5898 with ixekizumab, and no reactivations observed in pivotal trials of guselkumab, risankizumab, and tildrakizumab [14]. This low risk has been corroborated by the 2024 multicenter study by Torres et al., which evaluated 405 psoriasis patients with newly diagnosed LTBI who were treated with IL-17 or IL-23 inhibitors. Remarkably, only one TB reactivation (0.25%) occurred over a mean follow-up of 33 months, and 37.8% of patients did not receive full chemoprophylaxis [54].

Psoriasis in the setting of HIV infection often exhibits an atypical clinical course, characterized by increased severity, resistance to conventional treatments, and the potential for uncommon morphologic variants, including erythrodermic, rupioid, and palmoplantar forms. In some instances, the onset of severe psoriasis may herald previously undiagnosed HIV infection. Thus, HIV testing should be considered in patients with abrupt or unusually severe psoriasis presentations [55].

Management of psoriasis in HIV-positive patients demands a delicate balance between achieving disease control and minimizing further immunosuppression. Topical therapies and NB-UVB phototherapy remain first-line options, offering effective management without systemic immunologic compromise [56].

Systemic therapies must be selected cautiously. Methotrexate and cyclosporine, while effective for psoriasis, pose significant risks in HIV-positive patients due to their profound immunosuppressive effects. Their use should be reserved for cases where safer alternatives are unavailable, and only in patients with well-controlled HIV infection (CD4 counts >200 cells/μL and suppressed viral load under antiretroviral therapy). Even then, close monitoring for opportunistic infections is imperative [56].

Acitretin is considered a favorable systemic option for HIV-positive psoriasis patients. It is non-immunosuppressive, does not increase infection risk, and is particularly beneficial in hyperkeratotic variants of psoriasis, which are common in the context of HIV. However, its mucocutaneous side effects and impact on lipid metabolism must be weighed carefully [57].

Apremilast represents an excellent systemic treatment choice in HIV-positive individuals with psoriasis. It is not immunosuppressive, does not interact significantly with antiretroviral therapy, and has a favorable safety profile. Gastrointestinal side effects and mild weight loss are common but generally manageable [58].

Biologic agent therapy in HIV-positive patients is an evolving area. Emerging evidence suggests that TNF-α inhibitors, IL-17 inhibitors, and IL-23 inhibitors can be used cautiously in selected HIV-positive patients with well-controlled disease, particularly when other therapies fail. However, these cases should be managed collaboratively with infectious disease specialists. IL-17 and IL-23 inhibitors may be preferred over TNF-α inhibitors due to their more targeted immunomodulatory profiles and, theoretically, a lower impact on global immune surveillance [44].

In conclusion, psoriasis management in patients with latent tuberculosis or HIV infection necessitates rigorous screening, interdisciplinary coordination, and careful therapeutic selection. Topical therapies and NB-UVB phototherapy should be maximized for mild-to-moderate disease. For systemic therapy, IL-17 and IL-23 inhibitors, ustekinumab, and apremilast offer safe and effective options, while TNF-α inhibitors and conventional immunosuppressants must be used with caution or avoided. The primary goal is to achieve optimal disease control while minimizing infection risk and preserving immune function.

9. Inflammatory bowel disease

Psoriasis and inflammatory bowel disease (IBD) frequently coexist due to shared immunopathogenic mechanisms, especially involving the IL-23/Th17 axis. While some therapies are effective for both conditions, others—particularly IL-17 inhibitors—may increase the risk of IBD exacerbation or development [59]. Therefore, therapeutic selection in patients with concurrent psoriasis and inflammatory bowel disease requires careful consideration to balance dermatological effectiveness with gastrointestinal safety concerns optimally. Agents that are effective in both diseases, such as TNF-α inhibitors and IL-23 pathway inhibitors, are generally preferred, whereas therapies with the potential to worsen IBD must be avoided. A practical summary of treatment preferences based on IBD activity is presented in **Table 2**.

10. Malignancy

The presence of a current or previous malignancy, particularly lymphomas and skin cancers, significantly influences therapeutic decision-making in psoriasis management. In patients with a history of malignancy, topical therapies represent the safest initial treatment strategy. Emollients, corticosteroids, vitamin D analogs, and topical calcineurin inhibitors can be utilized without systemic immunosuppression. NB-UVB phototherapy is also considered safe in patients with a history of solid tumors or treated lymphoma, provided that prior skin cancer history is carefully considered [60]. In contrast, PUVA therapy should be avoided in individuals with a history of melanoma, multiple non-melanoma skin cancers (NMSCs), or significant actinic damage due to its mutagenic potential [61].

Among conventional systemic therapies, methotrexate warrants caution in the setting of malignancy. Long-term methotrexate use has been associated with an increased risk of lymphoproliferative disorders, particularly in patients positive for Epstein-Barr virus (EBV). Methotrexate-induced lymphomas may sometimes regress upon drug discontinuation, but reinitiation carries potential risk. Therefore, methotrexate is generally avoided in patients with active or recent lymphoma [62].

As a potent immunosuppressant, cyclosporine carries a well-established risk of NMSC and lymphomas, especially with prolonged use and in patients with prior ultraviolet exposure. Consequently, its use should be avoided in psoriasis patients with a history of cancer, except in short-term emergency situations under close oncologic monitoring [63]. Acitretin, in contrast, represents a favorable systemic option for psoriasis patients with prior malignancy as it exhibits chemopreventive effects against NMSC. Acitretin is particularly beneficial for psoriatic patients with a history of actinic keratoses, squamous cell carcinoma, or field cancerization, although its

IBD status	Preferred treatments	Treatments to consider carefully	Avoid	Supportive therapies
Active IBD [14]	• **TNF-α inhibitors** (adalimumab, infliximab) *(FDA-approved for Crohn and UC)*	• **Methotrexate** *(limited efficacy for IBD; mainly useful for joint symptoms)*	• **IL-17 inhibitors**	• Topical therapy
	• **Ustekinumab** *(FDA-approved for Crohn's disease)*			• NB-UVB
	• **Risankizumab** *(FDA-approved for Crohn's disease)*			
Controlled IBD [14]	• **Ustekinumab** *(FDA-approved for Crohn's disease)*	• **Tildrakizumab** *(psoriasis approved; limited data in IBD)*	• **IL-17 inhibitors**	• Topical therapy
	• **Risankizumab** *(FDA-approved for Crohn's disease)*	• **Tildrakizumab** *(psoriasis approved; limited data in IBD)*		• NB-UVB
	• **TNF-α inhibitors** (adalimumab, infliximab) *(FDA-approved for Crohn and UC)*	• **Apremilast** *(safe but no effect on IBD activity)*		
		• **Methotrexate** *(limited benefit)*		

Table 2.
Systemic treatment options for psoriasis with coexisting inflammatory bowel disease.

mucocutaneous side effects and teratogenicity must be managed appropriately [64]. Apremilast provides an additional safe systemic alternative. Its immunomodulatory effects are mild, and it has not been linked to an increased risk of malignancy in either clinical trials or real-world studies. It is especially advantageous for patients with a recent history of solid tumors or for those in whom conventional immunosuppressants are contraindicated [21].

TNF-α inhibitors have historically raised concern regarding malignancy risk, particularly for lymphoproliferative disorders [65]. While older meta-analyses yielded mixed results, recent large-scale data continue to support a cautious approach. A retrospective cohort study published in 2025 involving 7645 Korean patients with psoriasis and rheumatoid arthritis found no significant increase in the risk of common solid tumors—including colorectal, liver, lung, kidney, breast, and thyroid cancers—among TNF-α inhibitor users. However, the risk of lymphoma was significantly elevated in infliximab users, and leukemia risk increased in users of etanercept and adalimumab [66]. These findings reinforce current guideline recommendations to defer TNF-α inhibitor use for at least 5 years after remission in patients with a history of lymphoma or leukemia and to prefer other biologic classes when biological agent treatment is indicated [67].

IL-17 inhibitors, particularly secukinumab and ixekizumab, have demonstrated favorable safety profiles in patients with prior malignancy [68, 69]. Real-world case series and retrospective analyses of patients with various cancers treated with IL-17A inhibitors have shown no recurrence or progression during long-term follow-up periods [70]. This supports the cautious use of IL-17 blockers in psoriatic patients with a stable cancer history. Similarly, IL-23 inhibitors such as guselkumab and risankizumab have not been associated with malignancy recurrence in clinical trials or post-marketing data. These agents are increasingly considered safe and effective options in this clinical context [71]. Ustekinumab similarly exhibits a reassuring malignancy profile, with long-term follow-up data demonstrating no elevated cancer risk [14].

In conclusion, managing psoriasis in patients with a history of malignancy necessitates an individualized approach emphasizing oncologic safety. Topical therapies and NB-UVB phototherapy should be prioritized for mild disease. Among systemic options, acitretin, apremilast, and biologic agents targeting IL-17 or IL-23 pathways are preferred choices, offering effective disease control without compromising cancer surveillance. Multidisciplinary collaboration with oncology is essential to ensure that therapeutic strategies align with the patient's oncologic status and long-term health goals.

11. Psoriatic arthritis

Approximately 20–30% of patients with psoriasis will develop PsA during their lifetime, typically manifesting between the ages of 30 and 50 years. The pathogenesis of PsA shares common immunological pathways with cutaneous psoriasis, particularly involving the IL-23/Th17 axis, yet the clinical expression in musculoskeletal tissues necessitates specialized therapeutic strategies [11].

Early identification of PsA is critical to prevent irreversible joint damage and long-term disability. Screening questionnaires such as the Psoriasis Epidemiology Screening Tool (PEST) or the Toronto Psoriatic Arthritis Screen (ToPAS) can aid dermatologists in early detection. Diagnosis should be confirmed by rheumatologists based on the Classification Criteria for Psoriatic Arthritis (CASPAR) criteria, and treatment should be initiated promptly to prevent structural joint damage [72].

In cases of mild psoriasis and limited joint involvement, topical therapies and NB-UVB phototherapy may provide relief for cutaneous lesions, but they have no effect on joint inflammation. Therefore, systemic therapy is mandatory in PsA, regardless of the severity of cutaneous involvement, when arthritis is clinically evident [73]. A summarized treatment algorithm outlining the clinical approach to PsA management is presented in **Figure 2**.

In patients experiencing mild peripheral arthritis, NSAIDs and intra-articular corticosteroids can help alleviate symptoms. Methotrexate is often the first-line conventional synthetic DMARD (csDMARD), especially for peripheral arthritis. Nonetheless, its effectiveness in axial PsA, enthesitis, and dactylitis remains limited. Cyclosporine may provide quick symptom relief during severe PsA flare-ups but carries risks such as nephrotoxicity, hypertension, and metabolic issues. Due to these potential risks and the availability of biologic therapies, cyclosporine is now typically used only in rare, short-term indications. Apremilast presents a safe alternative in patients with mild disease or in those ineligible for biologic therapy, though its efficacy is modest compared to targeted biologics [19].

When csDMARDs are insufficient or when patients present with moderate-to-severe PsA, biologic DMARDs (bDMARDs) are the mainstay of treatment. TNF-α inhibitors, including adalimumab, etanercept, infliximab, certolizumab pegol, and golimumab, are the longest-established class of biologic agents used in the treatment of PsA. TNF-α inhibitors have demonstrated robust efficacy across all major clinical domains of PsA—including peripheral arthritis, axial involvement, enthesitis, and dactylitis. They are particularly effective in polyarticular peripheral arthritis, with pivotal trials such as RAPID-PsA, ADEPT, and GO-REVEAL showing significant improvements in both clinical remission and prevention of structural joint damage. In axial PsA, TNF-α inhibitors remain among the only biologics with proven efficacy,

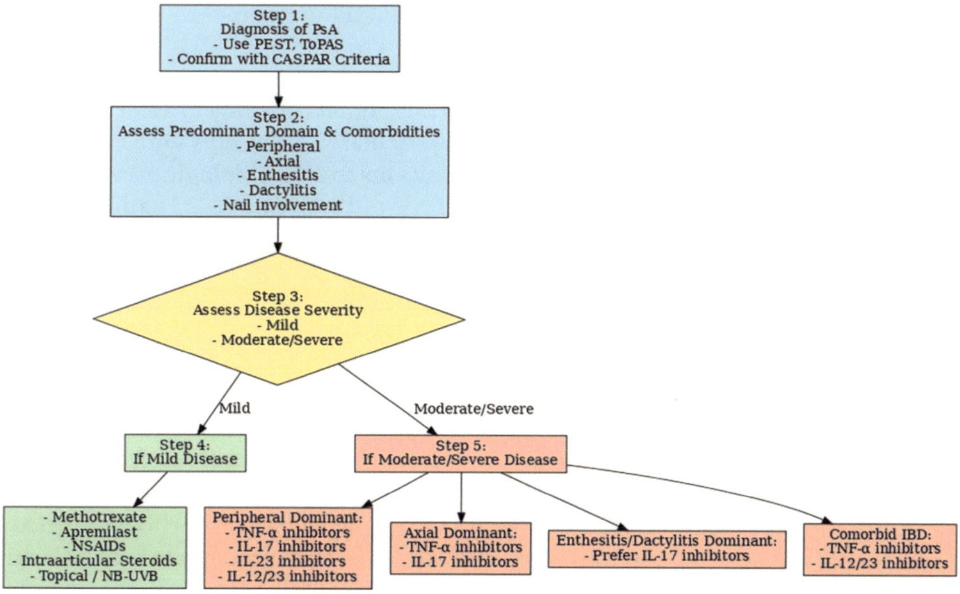

Figure 2.
Clinical treatment algorithm for the management of psoriatic arthritis.

reducing spinal inflammation and improving mobility, as validated by MRI and patient-reported outcomes [74].

IL-17 inhibitors, including secukinumab and ixekizumab, selectively block the IL-17A pathway and have demonstrated strong efficacy across multiple domains of PsA. These agents produce rapid and sustained clinical improvements in peripheral arthritis, enthesitis, dactylitis, and notably, axial disease [75]. In patients with axial PsA, secukinumab and ixekizumab significantly reduced spinal pain, morning stiffness, and MRI-confirmed inflammation. The phase 3 MAXIMISE trial specifically confirmed the efficacy of secukinumab in active sacroiliitis, reinforcing its value for axial involvement. Both agents have also been shown to achieve significant ACR20 response rates and inhibit radiographic progression over time [76].

Bimekizumab, a newer agent that targets both IL-17A and IL-17F, has further expanded the therapeutic landscape. In the BE OPTIMAL and BE COMPLETE phase 3 trials, bimekizumab demonstrated significantly greater efficacy than placebo in improving joint and cutaneous symptoms, achieving ACR50 rates of 44–46% and PASI100 responses in over 60% of patients by week 16. Importantly, bimekizumab showed superior efficacy in traditionally challenging domains such as enthesitis and dactylitis, with early onset of action. These data position IL-17 inhibitors as a potent option for comprehensive PsA management [77].

IL-23 inhibitors, such as guselkumab and risankizumab, have shown substantial efficacy in peripheral arthritis and skin disease, with emerging evidence supporting their potential benefit in enthesitis and dactylitis [78]. They demonstrated significant efficacy in joint involvement, with ACR20 response rates ranging from 57% to 64% in pivotal trials. Guselkumab, particularly at a dosing interval of every 4 weeks, was associated with superior inhibition of structural damage progression as measured by the van der Heijde-Sharp score compared to every 8-week dosing, placebo, and risankizumab. While both IL-23 inhibitors improved enthesitis and dactylitis outcomes, guselkumab demonstrated more consistent efficacy across multiple domains and trials, suggesting a potentially broader therapeutic impact in PsA disease phenotypes. However, their effectiveness in axial PsA is still under investigation, and current data suggest a less prominent role compared to TNF-α and IL-17 inhibitors in pure axial disease [79, 80].

Ustekinumab is effective for peripheral PsA, though its efficacy in axial disease is relatively lower. It remains a valuable option, particularly in patients with concomitant inflammatory bowel disease or contraindications to other biologic classes [73].

In conclusion, biologic therapies targeting TNF-α, IL-17, and IL-23 pathways have expanded the therapeutic arsenal and significantly improved patient outcomes. Optimal management demands careful consideration of the predominant disease domains, comorbidities, and long-term safety profiles of available agents, guided by current evidence-based recommendations.

12. Conclusion

Effective psoriasis management in special clinical contexts requires personalized, evidence-based strategies. Pregnancy and breastfeeding call for safer choices such as topical therapies, NB-UVB phototherapy, cyclosporine, and certolizumab pegol, while methotrexate and acitretin are contraindicated. Patients with hepatic or renal impairment benefit from IL-17 and IL-23 inhibitors due to favorable safety profiles. For those with congestive heart failure or demyelinating disease, IL-17 and IL-23 inhibitors are preferred over TNF-α inhibitors. Managing psoriasis in latent tuberculosis or HIV-positive patients necessitates rigorous screening and cautious therapy selection, favoring IL-17/IL-23 inhibitors, acitretin, and apremilast. In concurrent IBD, TNF-α and IL-23 inhibitors are optimal, whereas IL-17 inhibitors should be avoided. In patients with a history of malignancy, topical therapies, phototherapy, acitretin, apremilast, and IL-17 or IL-23 biologics are preferable due to their favorable safety profiles. Psoriatic arthritis treatment is effectively managed with biologics that target the TNF-α, IL-17, and IL-23 pathways. In conclusion, individualized and interdisciplinary approaches ensure optimal outcomes across these complex clinical scenarios.

Conflict of interest

The authors declare no conflict of interest.

Appendixes and nomenclature

PsA	psoriatic arthritis
NB-UVB	narrowband ultraviolet B phototherapy
PUVA	psoralen plus ultraviolet A phototherapy
TNF-α	tumor necrosis factor alpha
IL-17	interleukin-17
IL-23	interleukin-23
IL-12	interleukin-12
NMSC	non-melanoma skin cancer
CASPAR	classification criteria for psoriatic arthritis
PEST	psoriasis epidemiology screening tool
ToPAS	Toronto Psoriatic Arthritis Screen
IGRA	interferon-gamma release assay
TST	tuberculin skin test

Author details

Selda Pelin Kartal[1] and Tuğcan Yüksek[2]*

1 Health Sciences University, Ankara Elik City Hospital, Dermatology Clinic, Ankara, Turkey

2 Kyrenia Dr. Akcicek Government Hospital, Dermatology Clinic, Kyrenia, Northern Cyprus

*Address all correspondence to: tugcanyuksek6@gmail.com

References

[1] Murase JE, Heller MM, Butler DC. Safety of dermatologic medications in pregnancy and lactation: Part I. Pregnancy. Journal of the American Academy of Dermatology. 2014;**70**(3):401.e1-401.14; quiz 415

[2] Rose RF, Batchelor RJ, Turner D, Goulden V. Narrowband ultraviolet B phototherapy does not influence serum and red cell folate levels in patients with psoriasis. Journal of the American Academy of Dermatology. 2009;**61**(2):259-262

[3] El-Saie LT, Rabie AR, Kamel MI, Seddeik AK, Elsaie ML. Effect of narrowband ultraviolet B phototherapy on serum folic acid levels in patients with psoriasis. Lasers in Medical Science. 2011;**26**(4):481-485

[4] Vena GA, Cassano N, Bellia G, Colombo D. Psoriasis in pregnancy: Challenges and solutions. Psoriasis (Auckland, NZ). 2015;**5**:83-95

[5] Neema S, Kothari R, Rout A, Mani S, Bhatt S, Sandhu S. Systemic treatment of psoriasis in special population. Indian Journal of Dermatology, Venereology and Leprology. 2024;**90**(2):170-177

[6] Mariette X. Certolizumab, an anti-TNF safe during pregnancy? The CRIB Study results: An interview with Professor Xavier Mariette. Immunotherapy. 2017;**9**:793-795

[7] Johansen CB, Jimenez-Solem E, Haerskjold A, Sand FL, Thomsen SF. The use and safety of TNF inhibitors during pregnancy in women with psoriasis: A review. International Journal of Molecular Sciences. 2018;**19**(5):5

[8] Verberne EA, de Haan E, van Tintelen JP, Lindhout D, van Haelst MM. Fetal methotrexate syndrome: A systematic review of case reports. Reproductive Toxicology. 2019;**87**:125-139

[9] Heath MS, Sahni DR, Curry ZA, Feldman SR. Pharmacokinetics of tazarotene and acitretin in psoriasis. Expert Opinion on Drug Metabolism & Toxicology. 2018;**14**(9):919-927

[10] Balakirski G, Gerdes S, Beissert S, Ochsendorf F, von Kiedrowski R, Wilsmann-Theis D. Therapy of psoriasis during pregnancy and breast-feeding. JDDG - J Ger Soc Dermatology. 2022;**20**(5):653-683

[11] Yamazaki F. Psoriasis: Comorbidities. The Journal of Dermatology. 2021;**48**(6):732-740

[12] Nast A, Amelunxen L, Augustin M, Boehncke WH, Dressler C, Gaskins M, et al. S3 guideline for the treatment of psoriasis vulgaris, update—Short version part 2—Special patient populations and treatment situations. JDDG—Journal of the German Society of Dermatology. 2018;**16**(6):806-814

[13] Elmets CA, Leonardi CL, Davis DMR, Gelfand JM, Lichten J, Mehta NN, et al. Joint AAD-NPF guidelines of care for the management and treatment of psoriasis with awareness and attention to comorbidities. Journal of the American Academy of Dermatology. 2019;**80**(4):1073-1113. DOI: 10.1016/j.jaad.2018.11.058

[14] Lambert JLW, Segaert S, Ghislain PD, Hillary T, Nikkels A, Willaert F, et al. Practical recommendations for systemic treatment in psoriasis in case of coexisting inflammatory, neurologic, infectious or malignant disorders

(BETA-PSO: Belgian Evidence-based Treatment Advice in Psoriasis; part 2). Journal of the European Academy of Dermatology and Venereology. 2020;**34**(9):1914-1923

[15] Bellinato F, Maurelli M, Geat D, Girolomoni G, Gisondi P. Managing the patient with psoriasis and metabolic comorbidities. American Journal of Clinical Dermatology. 2024;**25**(4):527-540. DOI: 10.1007/s40257-024-00857-0

[16] Ting S-W, Chen Y-C, Huang Y-H. Risk of hepatitis B reactivation in patients with psoriasis on ustekinumab. Clinical Drug Investigation. 2018;**38**(9):873-880

[17] Kaushik SB, Lebwohl MG. Psoriasis: Which therapy for which patient: Focus on special populations and chronic infections. Journal of the American Academy of Dermatology. 2019;**80**(1):43-53

[18] Chiu H-Y, Hui RC-Y, Huang Y-H, Huang R-Y, Chen K-L, Tsai Y-C, et al. Safety profile of secukinumab in treatment of patients with psoriasis and concurrent hepatitis B or C: A multicentric prospective cohort study. Acta Dermato-Venereologica. 2018;**98**(9):829-834

[19] Nast A, Smith C, Spuls PI, Avila Valle G, Bata-Csörgö Z, Boonen H, et al. EuroGuiDerm guideline on the systemic treatment of psoriasis vulgaris—Part 2: Specific clinical and comorbid situations. Journal of the European Academy of Dermatology and Venereology. 2021;**35**(2):281-317

[20] Monks G. Psoriasis decision tree_2021. The Journal of Clinical and Aesthetic Dermatology. 2021;**14**(4):14-22

[21] Crowley J, Thaçi D, Joly P, Peris K, Papp KA, Goncalves J, et al. Long-term safety and tolerability of apremilast in patients with psoriasis: Pooled safety analysis for ≥156 weeks from 2 phase 3, randomized, controlled trials (ESTEEM 1 and 2). Journal of the American Academy of Dermatology. 2017;**77**(2):310-317.e1

[22] Pannu S, Rosmarin D. Psoriasis in patients with metabolic syndrome or type 2 diabetes mellitus: Treatment challenges. American Journal of Clinical Dermatology. 2021;**22**(3):293-300

[23] Elmets CA, Korman NJ, Prater EF, Wong EB, Rupani RN, Kivelevitch D, et al. Joint AAD–NPF guidelines of care for the management and treatment of psoriasis with topical therapy and alternative medicine modalities for psoriasis severity measures. Journal of the American Academy of Dermatology. 2021;**84**(2):432-470. DOI: 10.1016/j.jaad.2020.07.087

[24] Torres T, Puig L. Apremilast: A novel oral treatment for psoriasis and psoriatic arthritis. American Journal of Clinical Dermatology. 2018;**19**(1):23-32

[25] Stagakis I, Bertsias G, Karvounaris S, Kavousanaki M, Virla D, Raptopoulou A, et al. Anti-tumor necrosis factor therapy improves insulin resistance, beta cell function and insulin signaling in active rheumatoid arthritis patients with high insulin resistance. Arthritis Research & Therapy. 2012;**14**(3):R141

[26] Jiang W, Li Q, Zheng W. The impact of biologics targeting the IL-17 and IL-23 pathways on metabolic indicators in plaque psoriasis. Archives of Dermatological Research. 2025;**317**(1):643

[27] Zhang L, Wang Y, Qiu L, Wu J. Psoriasis and cardiovascular disease risk in European and East Asian populations: Evidence from meta-analysis and Mendelian randomization analysis. BMC Medicine. 2022;**20**(1):421

[28] Hugh J, Van Voorhees AS, Nijhawan RI, Bagel J, Lebwohl M, Blauvelt A, et al. From the Medical Board of the National Psoriasis Foundation: The risk of cardiovascular disease in individuals with psoriasis and the potential impact of current therapies. Journal of the American Academy of Dermatology. 2014;**70**(1):168-177

[29] Chen Y-J, Chang Y-T, Shen J-L, Chen T-T, Wang C-B, Chen C-M, et al. Association between systemic antipsoriatic drugs and cardiovascular risk in patients with psoriasis with or without psoriatic arthritis: A nationwide cohort study. Arthritis and Rheumatism. 2012;**64**(6):1879-1887

[30] Carretero G, Ribera M, Belinchón I, Carrascosa JM, Puig L, Ferrandiz C, et al. Guidelines for the use of acitretin in psoriasis. Actas Dermo-Sifiliográficas (English Edition). 2013;**104**(7):598-616

[31] Behnam SM, Behnam SE, Koo JY. TNF-alpha inhibitors and congestive heart failure. Skinmed. 2005;**4**(6): 363-368

[32] Chung ES, Packer M, Lo KH, Fasanmade AA, Willerson JT. Randomized, double-blind, placebo-controlled, pilot trial of infliximab, a chimeric monoclonal antibody to tumor necrosis factor-alpha, in patients with moderate-to-severe heart failure: Results of the anti-TNF Therapy Against Congestive Heart Failure (ATTACH) trial. Circulation. 2003;**107**(25):3133-3140

[33] Thatiparthi A, Martin A, Liu J, Egeberg A, Wu JJ. Biologic treatment algorithms for moderate-to-severe psoriasis with comorbid conditions and special populations: A review. American Journal of Clinical Dermatology. 2021;**22**(4):425-442

[34] Armstrong A, Paul C, Puig L, Boehncke WH, Freeman M, Torii H, et al. Safety of ixekizumab treatment for up to 5 years in adult patients with moderate-to-severe psoriasis: Results from greater than 17,000 patient-years of exposure. Dermatology and Therapy. 2020;**10**(1):133-150

[35] Bai F, Li GG, Liu Q, Niu X, Li R, Ma H. Short-term efficacy and safety of IL-17, IL-12/23, and IL-23 inhibitors brodalumab, secukinumab, ixekizumab, ustekinumab, guselkumab, tildrakizumab, and risankizumab for the treatment of moderate to severe plaque psoriasis: A systematic review and network. Journal of Immunology Research. 2019;**2019**:2546161

[36] Langley RG, Lebwohl M, Krueger GG, Szapary PO, Wasfi Y, Chan D, et al. Long-term efficacy and safety of ustekinumab, with and without dosing adjustment, in patients with moderate-to-severe psoriasis: Results from the PHOENIX 2 study through 5 years of follow-up. The British Journal of Dermatology. 2015;**172**(5):1371-1383

[37] Navarro-Compán V, Puig L, Vidal S, Ramírez J, Llamas-Velasco M, Fernández-Carballido C, et al. The paradigm of IL-23-independent production of IL-17F and IL-17A and their role in chronic inflammatory diseases. Frontiers in Immunology. 2023;**14**:1191782

[38] Charlton O, Phan K, Smith SD, Parratt J. Psoriasis in family members of patients with multiple sclerosis. Multiple Sclerosis and Related Disorders. 2019;**36**:101421

[39] Liu M, Huang YYM, Hsu S, Kass JS. Neurological and neuropsychiatric adverse effects of dermatologic medications. CNS Drugs. 2016;**30**(12): 1149-1168

[40] Ellis CN, Fradin MS, Messana JM, Brown MD, Siegel MT, Hartley AH, et al. Cyclosporine for plaque-type psoriasis. Results of a multidose, double-blind trial. The New England Journal of Medicine. 1991;**324**(5):277-284

[41] Takeno M. Positioning of apremilast in treatment of Behçet's disease. Modern Rheumatology. 2020;**30**(2):219-224

[42] Kemanetzoglou E, Andreadou E. CNS demyelination with TNF-α blockers. Current Neurology and Neuroscience Reports. 2017;**17**(4):36

[43] Boggs JME, Barnes L. Demyelination during anti-tumour necrosis factor therapy for psoriasis. Clinical and Experimental Dermatology. 2018;**43**(5):577-578

[44] Gisondi P, Fargnoli MC, Amerio P, Argenziano G, Bardazzi F, Bianchi L, et al. Italian adaptation of EuroGuiDerm guideline on the systemic treatment of chronic plaque psoriasis. Italian Journal of Dermatology and Venereology. 2022;**157**(1):1-78

[45] Havrdová E, Belova A, Goloborodko A, Tisserant A, Wright A, Wallstroem E, et al. Activity of secukinumab, an anti-IL-17A antibody, on brain lesions in RRMS: Results from a randomized, proof-of-concept study. Journal of Neurology. 2016;**263**(7):1287-1295

[46] Herrera-Acosta E, Garriga-Martina GG, Suárez-Pérez JA, Martínez-García EA, Herrera-Ceballos E. Ixekizumab for patients with plaque psoriasis affected by multiple sclerosis: Case report. Sultan Qaboos University Medical Journal. 2021;**21**(3):488-490

[47] Chang S, Chambers CJ, Liu F-T, Armstrong AW. Successful treatment of psoriasis with ustekinumab in patients with multiple sclerosis. Dermatology Online Journal. 2015;**21**(7):3

[48] Gordon KB, Strober B, Lebwohl M, Augustin M, Blauvelt A, Poulin Y, et al. Efficacy and safety of risankizumab in moderate-to-severe plaque psoriasis (UltIMMa-1 and UltIMMa-2): Results from two double-blind, randomised, placebo-controlled and ustekinumab-controlled phase 3 trials. Lancet (London, England). 2018;**392**(10148):650-661

[49] Reich K, Armstrong AW, Foley P, Song M, Wasfi Y, Randazzo B, et al. Efficacy and safety of guselkumab, an anti-interleukin-23 monoclonal antibody, compared with adalimumab for the treatment of patients with moderate to severe psoriasis with randomized withdrawal and retreatment: Results from the phase III, double-blind, placebo- and active comparator-controlled VOYAGE 2 trial. Journal of the American Academy of Dermatology. 2017;**76**(3):418-431

[50] Martínez-López A, Rodriguez-Granger J, Ruiz-Villaverde R. Screening for latent tuberculosis in the patient with moderate to severe psoriasis who is a candidate for systemic and/or biologic therapy. Actas Dermo-Sifiliográficas. 2016;**107**(3):207-214

[51] Cantini F, Niccoli L, Capone A, Petrone L, Goletti D. Risk of tuberculosis reactivation associated with traditional disease modifying anti-rheumatic drugs and non-anti-tumor necrosis factor biologics in patients with rheumatic disorders and suggestion for clinical practice. Expert Opinion on Drug Safety. 2019;**18**(5):415-425

[52] Tsai T-F, Ho V, Song M, Szapary P, Kato T, Wasfi Y, et al. The safety of ustekinumab treatment in patients with moderate-to-severe psoriasis

and latent tuberculosis infection. The British Journal of Dermatology. 2012;**167**(5):1145-1152

[53] Zheng Y, Gao XJ, Huang JJ, Chen XM, Liao Y, Liu JM, et al. The safety assessment of ustekinumab on psoriasis and psoriatic arthritis: A real-world analysis based on the FDA adverse event reporting system database. International Immunopharmacology. 2025;**151**:114339. DOI: 10.1016/j.intimp.2025.114339

[54] Torres T, Chiricozzi A, Puig L, Lé AM, Marzano AV, Dapavo P, et al. Treatment of psoriasis patients with latent tuberculosis using IL-17 and IL-23 inhibitors: A retrospective, multinational, multicentre study. American Journal of Clinical Dermatology. 2024;**25**(2):333-342. DOI: 10.1007/s40257-024-00845-4

[55] Ceccarelli M, Venanzi Rullo E, Vaccaro M, Facciolà A, d'Aleo F, Paolucci IA, et al. HIV-associated psoriasis: Epidemiology, pathogenesis, and management. Dermatologic Therapy. 2019;**32**(2):e12806

[56] Jugovac V, Gulin M, Barić D, Drvar DL, Čeović R. Treatment of plaque-psoriasis in HIV-positive patients. Acta Dermatovenerologica Alpina, Pannonica et Adriatica. 2024;**33**(1):37-40

[57] Menon K, Van Voorhees AS, Bebo BFJ, Gladman DD, Hsu S, Kalb RE, et al. Psoriasis in patients with HIV infection: From the medical board of the National Psoriasis Foundation. Journal of the American Academy of Dermatology. 2010;**62**(2):291-299

[58] Megna M, Lauletta G, Tommasino N, Salsano A, Battista T, Ruggiero A, et al. Management of psoriasis patients with serious infectious diseases. Advances in Therapy. 2024;**41**(6):2099-2111

[59] Fieldhouse KA, Ukaibe S, Crowley EL, Khanna R, O'Toole A, Gooderham MJ. Inflammatory bowel disease in patients with psoriasis treated with interleukin-17 inhibitors. Drugs in Context. 2020;**9**:2020-2-1. DOI: 10.7573/dic.2020-2-1

[60] Naldi L. Malignancy concerns with psoriasis treatments using phototherapy, methotrexate, cyclosporin, and biologics: Facts and controversies. Clinics in Dermatology. 2010;**28**(1):88-92

[61] Morison WL, Baughman RD, Day RM, Forbes PD, Hoenigsmann H, Krueger GG, et al. Consensus workshop on the toxic effects of long-term PUVA therapy. Archives of Dermatology. 1998;**134**(5):595-598

[62] Afonso C, Roque A, Almeida C, Pimentão MB, Julião MJ, Silva R, et al. Methotrexate-associated lymphoproliferative disorder in a patient with psoriasis: A case report and review of the literature. Case Reports in Hematology. 2022;**2022**:7178065

[63] Paul CF, Ho VC, McGeown C, Christophers E, Schmidtmann B, Guillaume J-C, et al. Risk of malignancies in psoriasis patients treated with cyclosporine: A 5 y cohort study. The Journal of Investigative Dermatology. 2003;**120**(2):211-216

[64] Pang M-L, Murase JE, Koo J. An updated review of acitretin—A systemic retinoid for the treatment of psoriasis. Expert Opinion on Drug Metabolism & Toxicology. 2008;**4**(7):953-964

[65] Geller S, Xu H, Lebwohl M, Nardone B, Lacouture ME, Kheterpal M. Malignancy risk and recurrence with psoriasis and its treatments: A concise update. American Journal of Clinical Dermatology. 2018;**19**(3):363-375

[66] Song J, Kim SR, Kim Y-J, Park SJ, Jeong S, Park SM. Risk of hematologic malignancies in psoriasis and rheumatoid arthritis patients using long term TNF-α inhibitors: A retrospective nationwide study. Scientific Reports. 2025;**15**(1):7949

[67] Smith CH, Jabbar-Lopez ZK, Yiu ZZ, Bale T, Burden AD, Coates LC, et al. British Association of Dermatologists guidelines for biologic therapy for psoriasis 2017. The British Journal of Dermatology. 2017;**177**(3):628-636

[68] Pellegrini C, Esposito M, Rossi E, Gisondi P, Piaserico S, Dapavo P, et al. Secukinumab in patients with psoriasis and a personal history of malignancy: A multicenter real-life observational study. Dermatology and Therapy. 2022;**12**(11):2613-2626

[69] Deodhar A, Blauvelt A, Lebwohl M, Feely M, Kronbergs A, Eberhart N, et al. Long-term safety of Ixekizumab in adults with psoriasis, psoriatic arthritis, or axial spondyloarthritis: A post-hoc analysis of final safety data from 25 randomized clinical trials. Arthritis Research & Therapy. 2024;**26**(1):49

[70] Mastorino L, Dapavo P, Avallone G, Merli M, Cariti C, Rubatto M, et al. Biologic treatment for psoriasis in cancer patients: Should they still be considered forbidden? The Journal of Dermatological Treatment. 2022;**33**(5):2495-2502

[71] Wu S, Xu Y, Yang L, Guo L, Jiang X. Short-term risk and long-term incidence rate of infection and malignancy with IL-17 and IL-23 inhibitors in adult patients with psoriasis and psoriatic arthritis: A systematic review and meta-analysis. Frontiers in Immunology. 2023;**14**:1294416

[72] Başkan EB. Treatment algorithms for special cases. TURKDERM - Turkish Archives of Dermatology and Venereology. 2022;**56**(Suppl 1):80-85

[73] Atakan N, Gürer M, Onsun N, Özarmağan G. Updated Turkish guidelines for the management of psoriasis with biologic agents. TURKDERM - Turkish Archives of Dermatology and Venereology. 2010;**44**:105-112

[74] Lubrano E, Scriffignano S, Perrotta FM. TNF-alpha inhibitors for the six treatment targets of psoriatic arthritis. Expert Review of Clinical Immunology. 2019;**15**(12):1303-1312

[75] Gossec L, Kerschbaumer A, Ferreira RJO, Aletaha D, Baraliakos X, Bertheussen H, et al. EULAR recommendations for the management of psoriatic arthritis with pharmacological therapies: 2023 update. Annals of the Rheumatic Diseases. 2024;**83**(6):706-719

[76] Baraliakos X, Gossec L, Pournara E, Jeka S, Mera-Varela A, D'Angelo S, et al. Secukinumab in patients with psoriatic arthritis and axial manifestations: Results from the double-blind, randomised, phase 3 MAXIMISE trial. Annals of the Rheumatic Diseases. 2021;**80**(5):582-590

[77] Merola JF, Landewé R, McInnes IB, Mease PJ, Ritchlin CT, Tanaka Y, et al. Bimekizumab in patients with active psoriatic arthritis and previous inadequate response or intolerance to tumour necrosis factor-α inhibitors: A randomised, double-blind, placebo-controlled, phase 3 trial (BE COMPLETE). Lancet (London, England). 2023;**401**(10370):38-48

[78] Kerschbaumer A, Smolen JS, Ferreira RJO, Bertheussen H, Baraliakos X, Aletaha D, et al. Efficacy and safety of pharmacological treatment of psoriatic arthritis: A systematic literature research informing the 2023 update of the EULAR recommendations

for the management of psoriatic arthritis. Annals of the Rheumatic Diseases. 2024;**83**(6):760-774

[79] Mease PJ, Rahman P, Gottlieb AB, Kollmeier AP, Hsia EC, Xu XL, et al. Guselkumab in biologic-naive patients with active psoriatic arthritis (DISCOVER-2): A double-blind, randomised, placebo-controlled phase 3 trial. Lancet (London, England). 2020;**395**(10230):1126-1136

[80] Kristensen LE, Keiserman M, Papp K, McCasland L, White D, Lu W, et al. Efficacy and safety of risankizumab for active psoriatic arthritis: 24-week results from the randomised, double-blind, phase 3 KEEPsAKE 1 trial. Annals of the Rheumatic Diseases. 2022;**81**(2):225-231

Chapter 4

Paradoxical Reactions to Biologic Therapies in Patients with Plaque Psoriasis

Mihaela Georgescu, Maria Magdalena Constantin, Mădălina Mariana Motoacă and Daniel O. Costache

Abstract

Paradoxical psoriasis has been reported since 2003–2005. It is characterized by its occurrence independently of the underlying disease or the type of anti-TNF agent used, and it resolves once the treatment is discontinued. Unlike de novo psoriasis, paradoxical psoriasis is considered a side effect of TNF blockade. The pathophysiological mechanism involves an imbalance between TNF and type 1 IFN. The onset of skin manifestations can vary, ranging from 1 month to 10 years, with an average of 16.4 months. Approximately 2–5% of patients treated with TNF-alpha inhibitors develop paradoxical psoriasis. Females, particularly those with a personal or family history of inflammatory skin diseases, are more commonly affected. In addition, IL-17 and IL-23 inhibitors have been associated with worsening psoriasis, often triggering flares with altered psoriasis morphology.

Keywords: paradoxical reactions, psoriasis, pustular psoriasis, anti-TNF alfa, anti-Il17

1. Introduction

1.1 Working hypothesis, and specific objectives

Paradoxical psoriasis represents a distinct clinical entity that has been documented since the early 2000s, with initial reports dating back to 2003 [1] and 2005 [2]. Unlike classical psoriasis, paradoxical psoriasis emerges independently of the underlying disease or the specific type of anti-tumor necrosis factor (TNF) agent administered and typically resolves following drug discontinuation. As such, it is not considered a manifestation of *de novo* psoriasis but rather an adverse reaction directly associated with TNF-α inhibition.

The underlying pathophysiological mechanism is thought to stem from an imbalance between tumor necrosis factor (TNF) and type I interferons (IFNs) [3]. Specifically, psoriasiform eruptions are triggered by the suppression of TNF-α signaling, which diminishes the TNF-α–mediated negative feedback on plasmacytoid dendritic cells (pDCs). This results in the excessive production of type I IFNs, particularly IFN-α [4]. TNF-α normally acts to inhibit the maturation of pDCs and suppress IFN-α secretion. Its inhibition, therefore, leads to dysregulated IFN-α production, which subsequently contributes to the development of psoriatic lesions.

Histopathological studies of skin affected by plaque psoriasis have revealed elevated IFN-α expression within vascular and perivascular dermal lymphocytic infiltrates [5]. Another proposed mechanism involves the immune modulation associated with TNF-α blockade: an increase in T helper 17 (Th17) cells, a decrease in regulatory T cells (Tregs), and enhanced interleukin-22 (IL-22) production. IL-22, in turn, exerts pro-inflammatory effects on keratinocytes, sustaining the psoriatic process [6].

Emerging evidence also highlights the role of skin dysbiosis in the pathogenesis of paradoxical psoriasis. Alterations in the skin microbiome's composition and function may represent critical factors contributing to disease onset and progression [7].

The latency period for the appearance of cutaneous manifestations varies widely, ranging from 1 month to as long as 10 years, with an average onset of approximately 16.4 months following initiation of TNF-α inhibitor therapy [4]. Paradoxical psoriasis affects an estimated 2–5% of patients receiving TNF-α blockers [8], with a higher prevalence observed in females, particularly those with a personal or familial history of inflammatory skin conditions [7].

Beyond TNF-α inhibitors, other biologic agents have also been implicated in paradoxical psoriatic reactions. IL-17 inhibitors may induce morphological changes in psoriatic lesions or provoke new eruptions [4], while IL-23 inhibitors have also been reported as potential triggers of paradoxical psoriasis [9].

2. Objectives

The primary objective of this chapter is to describe and analyze cases of paradoxical reactions associated with biologic therapies administered to patients diagnosed with plaque psoriasis.

3. Patients and methods

A retrospective study was conducted involving patients diagnosed with plaque psoriasis who were undergoing biologic therapy, including anti-TNF-α agents (infliximab, adalimumab, certolizumab pegol, and etanercept), anti-interleukin agents (anti-IL-17: secukinumab and ixekizumab; anti-IL-23: risankizumab, guselkumab, and tildrakizumab; and anti-IL-12/23: ustekinumab), and phosphodiesterase-4 (PDE4) inhibitors (apremilast). The patients were recruited from the Dermatology Department 2 of Colentina Clinical Hospital and the Central Military Emergency University Hospital "Dr. Carol Davila" in Bucharest, covering the period from 2008 to 2023.

Clinical and demographic data were collected, including

- Sex (male or female)
- Age
- Area of residence (urban or rural)

- Type and class of biologic therapy (anti-TNF-α [infliximab, adalimumab, certolizumab pegol, and etanercept], anti-IL-17 [secukinumab and ixekizumab], anti-IL-23 [risankizumab, guselkumab, and tildrakizumab], anti-IL-12/23 [ustekinumab], PDE4 inhibitor [apremilast])

- Number of biologic therapies per patient

- Number of treatment switches per patient

- Presence of comorbidities.

For patients enrolled in the National Program for Biologic Therapy, data were collected using clinical and laboratory documentation from Annex 3 and the Romanian Registry for Dermatological Treatments (SRD).

3.1 Inclusion criteria

- Confirmed diagnosis of plaque psoriasis

- Signed informed consent for medical procedures and publishing (including consent for clinical photography)

- Fulfillment of the national protocol for initiating biologic therapy (PASI >10 and DLQI >10).

3.2 Exclusion criteria

- Refusal to provide informed consent for medical procedures.

4. Results

4.1 Case 1

The first case was published. We present the case of a 55-year-old female patient diagnosed with spondyloarthritis since 2018. She had a mixed form of spondyloarthritis, positive for the HLA-B27 gene. She was prescribed secukinumab (IL-17a inhibitor), but after 6 months of treatment, she developed a bilateral pustular eruption. The clinical diagnosis of pustular psoriasis was confirmed by a biopsy. The eruption was classified as a paradoxical drug reaction to an IL-17a inhibitor. The patient underwent a switch of treatment, the chosen drug being guselkumab [10].

4.2 Case 2

A 62-year-old female patient with a known history of plaque psoriasis since the age of 18—histopathologically confirmed in 2019—developed a new eruption approximately 12 months after initiating treatment with ixekizumab. The eruption was characterized by erythematous-squamous plaques with superficial pustules localized to the palms and soles (**Figure 1**). The patient had previously undergone topical treatment with isoconazole nitrate cream for six weeks, with no clinical improvement.

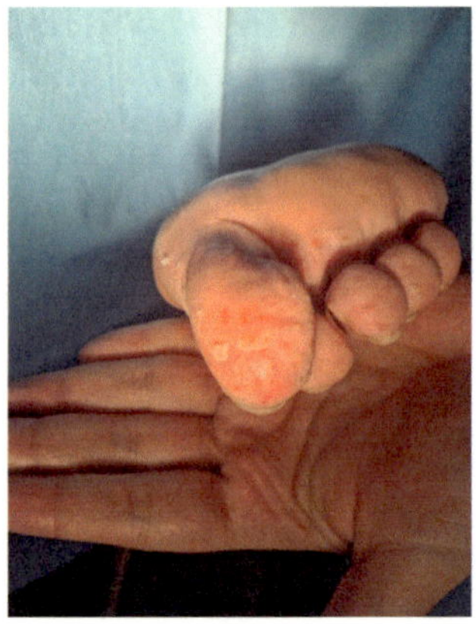

Figure 1.
Clinical presentation—erythematous, scaly plaques with superficial pustules on the right hallux (personal archive).

A diagnosis of paradoxical reaction was established, specifically pustular-type psoriasis vulgaris. A skin biopsy was performed on a lesion located on the dorsal surface of the right foot (**Figure 2**). Histopathological examination confirmed the diagnosis of plaque psoriasis (**Figures 3** and **4**).

Systemic treatment with methotrexate was initiated at a dose of 15 mg/week for 10 months, in combination with narrowband UVB (TL01) phototherapy administered three times per week, totaling 25 sessions. Clinically, the patient experienced alternating periods of remission and relapse. Consequently, a therapeutic switch to guselkumab was made while continuing methotrexate for an additional three months.

4.3 Case 3

A 34-year-old female patient, known to have plaque psoriasis since 2015, was undergoing treatment with a biosimilar of infliximab for 5.5 months when she presented in 2017 to the Clinical Dermatology Department, Central Military Emergency University Hospital "Dr. Carol Davila," Bucharest. She reported the onset of a new

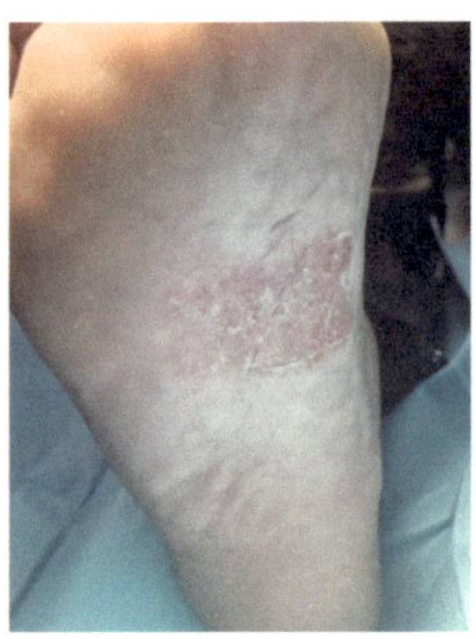

Figure 2.
Clinical presentation—erythematous, scaly plaques with superficial pustules on the right plantar surface (personal archive).

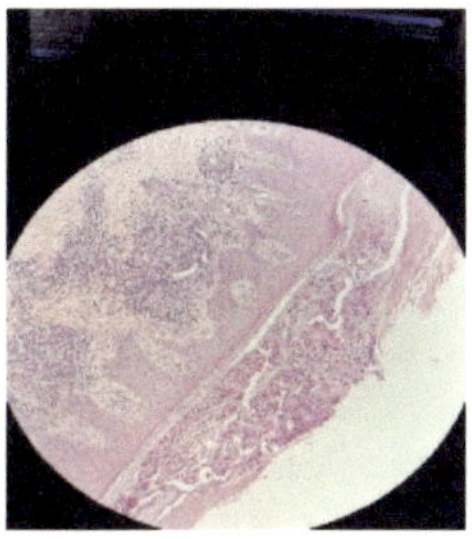

Figure 3.
Histopathological aspect—regular acanthosis of the epidermis, elongation of rete ridges, areas of hypogranulosis alternating with hypergranulosis, parakeratosis, horn and intraepithelial microabscesses, lymphoplasmacytic inflammatory infiltrate predominantly perivascular, and dilated capillaries in the superficial dermis (hematoxylin and eosin stain) (personal archive).

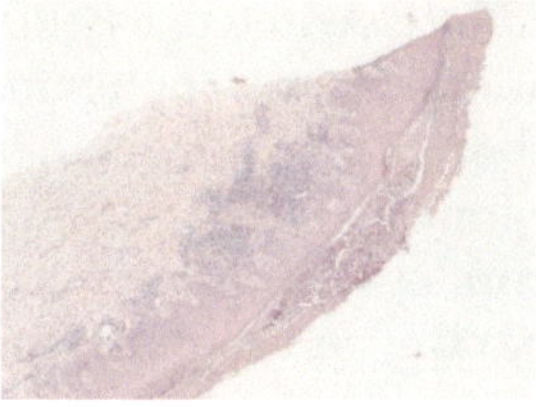

Figure 4.
Histological image, 10× magnification—plaque psoriasis (personal archive).

skin eruption approximately six weeks prior, characterized by erythematous-squamous plaques and large patches located on the palms and soles, with occasional pustules on the plantar surfaces (**Figure 5**).

Clinical examination revealed widespread erythematous plaques with peripheral scaling, irregular in shape and poorly demarcated, involving the entire body. According to her medical history, she had received systemic corticosteroid therapy (two 16 mg tablets per day) since the eruption began, without significant clinical improvement.

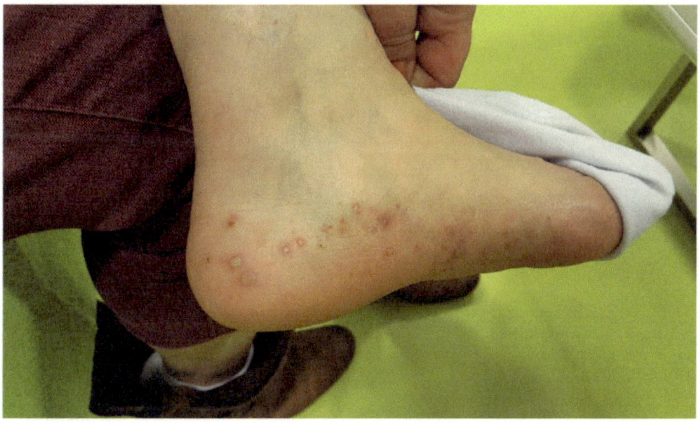

Figure 5.
Clinical presentation—erythematous-squamous plaques on the left foot (personal archive).

Her personal medical history included chronic autoimmune thyroiditis, virilization syndrome, ovarian dystrophy, hirsutism, obesity, and hypomagnesemia. Laboratory investigations were within normal limits, except for low serum magnesium levels. Both the abdominopelvic ultrasound and chest X-ray revealed no pathological findings.

4.4 Case 4

A 63-year-old female patient with a known diagnosis of plaque psoriasis since 2012, confirmed histopathologically in 2016, presented in November 2019 with erythroderma, occurring two months after initiation of secukinumab therapy (fifth loading dose pen-injector). The presumptive diagnosis was generalized paradoxical pustular psoriasis following IL-17a inhibitor therapy (**Figures 6** and 7).

According to the patient's history, she had been previously treated with etanercept between 2012 and 2018, followed by a switch to ustekinumab from 2018 until July 2019. Upon presentation, the patient underwent hemodynamic stabilization and was initiated on treatment with methotrexate (15 mg/week for 3 months) and systemic corticosteroids (methylprednisolone 0.5 mg/kg/day for 1 month).

Three months after the erythrodermic episode, she was reintroduced into the National Biological Therapy Program, and adalimumab treatment was initiated in 2020. The patient remains on this therapy to date.

Relevant comorbidities included morbid obesity (BMI = 42.8 kg/m^2), psoriatic arthritis, depressive syndrome, type 2 diabetes mellitus, and essential hypertension.

The following three patients developed palmoplantar eruptions after initiating the new citrate-free formulation of ixekizumab:

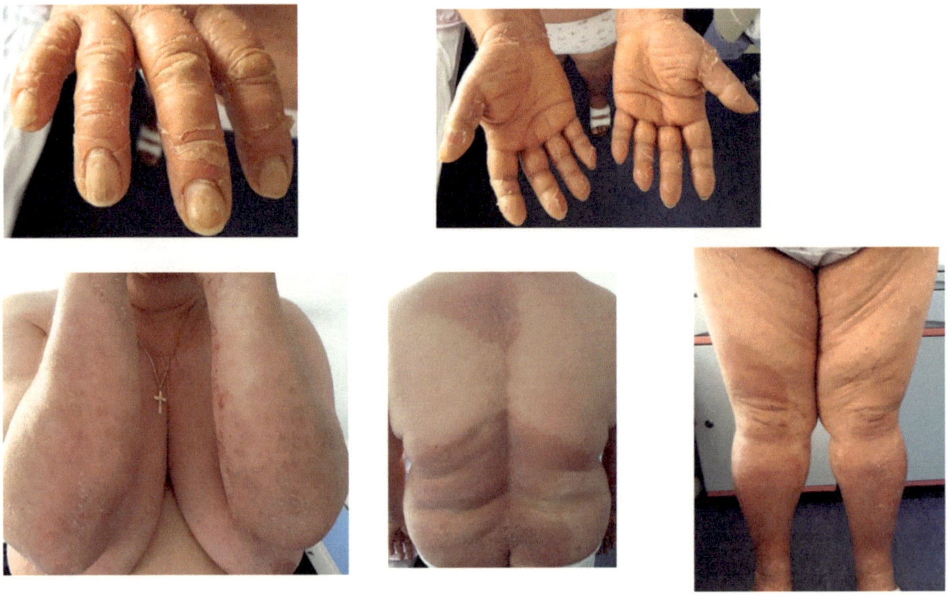

Figure 6.
Generalized clinical presentation (personal archive).

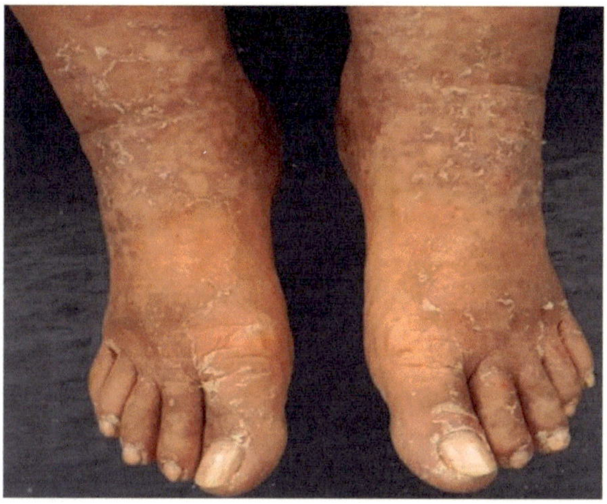

Figure 7.
Close-up view—pustular lesions on erythematous-squamous plaques, located on the soles and lower legs (personal archive).

4.5 Case 5

A 48-year-old overweight female patient (BMI = 26 kg/m^2), known to have had chronic plaque psoriasis since 2021, histopathologically confirmed in 2022, developed a palmoplantar eruption during treatment with the citrate-free formulation of ixekizumab (**Figure 8**). This was her second line of innovative therapy; the first was apremilast, administered between May and November 2022, which proved ineffective. Following the onset of the eruption, treatment with methotrexate at a dose of 15 mg/week was initiated for 3 months, leading to progressive improvement and complete resolution of skin lesions after 6 months.

Relevant medical history included cervical spondylodiscoarthrosis with left-sided rachialgia, left scapulohumeral periarthritis with impingement syndrome, tendon calcifications, and psoriatic arthropathy.

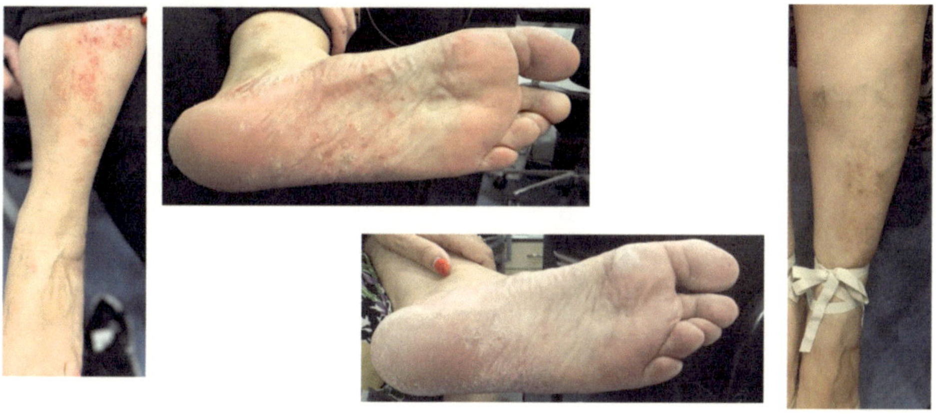

Figure 8.
Clinical presentation—pustular lesions on the plantar surface (Personal archive).

4.6 Case 6

A 40-year-old male patient with normal body weight (BMI = 20.3 kg/m^2), diagnosed with chronic plaque psoriasis since 2006 and confirmed histopathologically in 2017 was initiated on biologic therapy with ixekizumab in April 2019. In 2023, after switching to the citrate-free formulation of ixekizumab, he developed a new palmoplantar psoriatic eruption (**Figures 9** and **10**). In addition, the patient presented with psoriatic nail involvement.

The eruption improved with the use of topical corticosteroids, while the patient continued treatment with the citrate-free formulation.

4.7 Case 7

A 59-year-old female, diagnosed with vulgar psoriasis since 1992, histopathologically confirmed in 2021, was initiated on ixekizumab therapy in November 2022. The patient developed a palmoplantar eruption of vulgar psoriasis after switching to the citrate-free formulation of ixekizumab. She underwent topical dermatocorticosteroid treatment, leading to remission of the eruption within 6 months. However, the patient was switched to adalimumab biosimilar treatment in May 2023.

Personal medical history: Psoriatic arthritis with peripheral involvement, dyslipidemia, uterine fibromatosis, carpal tunnel syndrome, ischemic heart disease, and bilateral carotid atherosclerosis. Notably, scalp involvement was also observed.

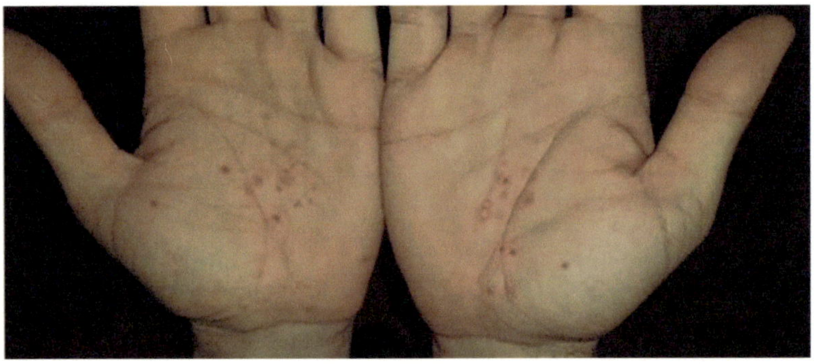

Figure 9.
Clinical detail—palmar eruption (Personal archive).

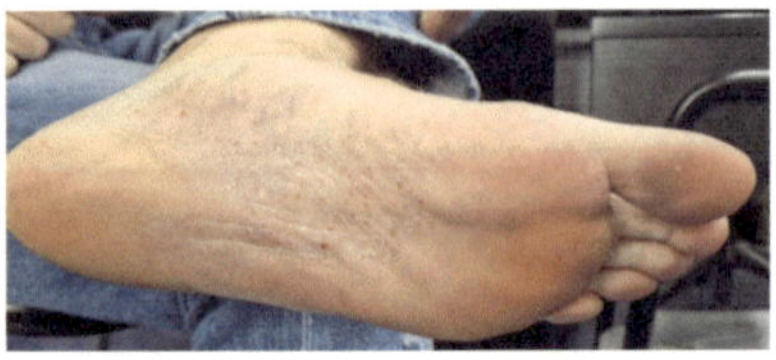

Figure 10.
Clinical detail—plantar eruption (Personal archive).

DOI: http://dx.doi.org/10.5772/intechopen.1011589

5. Discussions

The largest study on paradoxical reactions in patients treated with TNF inhibitors included 30 patients. The reactions observed included psoriasis (generalized plaques and palmoplantar pustulosis), alopecia, and neutrophilic dermatitis. Among TNF inhibitors, adalimumab was the most frequently reported, followed by infliximab. Regarding treatment switches, patients who switched to another anti-TNF did not achieve complete remission, while only a small proportion of those who switched to a different class of therapeutic agents achieved partial resolution [11]. From the cases we reported, only one case involved a paradoxical reaction, specifically with an infliximab biosimilar.

Generalized pustular psoriasis (GPP) represents a rare and severe subtype of pustular psoriasis, clinically distinct from plaque psoriasis, and characterized by widespread pustular eruptions accompanied by systemic symptoms resembling sepsis. The condition displays a female predominance, with a mean age of onset around 31 years, lower than that observed in palmoplantar pustular psoriasis (PPP) or acrodermatitis continua of Hallopeau, which typically manifests around the age of 44.

While plaque psoriasis is primarily mediated by the adaptive immune system through the IL-17/IL-23 axis, pustular variants, particularly GPP, involve hyperactivation of the innate immune response. A pivotal role is played by the IL-36 cytokine pathway, which stimulates keratinocytes to produce IL-23 and TNF-α, consequently enhancing Th17 cell proliferation and promoting elevated IL-17 expression.

Recent advances in molecular genetics have revealed a likely monogenic background for pustular psoriasis, as evidenced by mutations in three key genes of the innate cutaneous immune system: IL36RN, CARD14, and AP1S3. These findings support the classification proposed by the European Rare and Severe Psoriasis Expert Network (ERASPEN), which recognizes pustular psoriasis as a heterogeneous disease entity with three major subtypes: generalized pustular psoriasis, palmoplantar pustulosis, and acrodermatitis continua of Hallopeau.

The acute form of GPP, often referred to as von Zumbusch psoriasis, is marked by the sudden onset of pustules, fever, and systemic malaise, which can pose diagnostic and therapeutic challenges. No definitive cure is currently available for GPP, and relapses are common, necessitating long-term disease management.

Palmoplantar pustular psoriasis (PPP), in particular, is notorious for its therapeutic resistance. First-line treatment typically involves topical agents; however, systemic therapies are considered in patients unresponsive to local modalities. Therapeutic options include cyclosporine, oral retinoids, and oral PUVA, either as monotherapy or in combination (e.g., retinoid-PUVA). Despite their use, the majority of clinical data stem from case reports, retrospective analyses, and expert consensus rather than randomized controlled trials.

Recent studies have explored the role of biologic agents in PPP. Among these, guselkumab, an anti-IL-23 monoclonal antibody, has shown promising results in Japanese populations, with significant improvements in the Palmoplantar Pustulosis Area and Severity Index (PPPASI), Palmoplantar Pustulosis Severity Index (PPSI), and Dermatology Life Quality Index (DLQI). Currently, guselkumab is approved for PPP treatment exclusively in Japan.

Another emerging therapeutic option is spesolimab, a monoclonal antibody targeting IL-36. In clinical trials, spesolimab demonstrated a $\geq 50\%$ reduction in PPPASI scores by week 16 in 32% of patients receiving either 300 or 900 mg doses.

IL-17 inhibitors—such as secukinumab, ixekizumab, and brodalumab—have also been investigated in pustular variants. However, their effectiveness varies. The 2PRECISE trial reported a 75% PPPASI reduction in only 41.8% of patients treated with secukinumab 300 mg/month by week 52. Comparative analyses suggest that ixekizumab may outperform secukinumab in PPP management, based on both PPPASI improvements and patient-reported quality of life scores (DLQI).

IL-17 inhibitors, while generally well tolerated, may induce adverse events including injection site reactions, upper respiratory tract infections, oral candidiasis, and conjunctivitis. Moreover, paradoxical pustular psoriasis has been documented in patients receiving anti-TNF or IL-17 therapies, manifesting as palmoplantar pustular flares or acrodermatitis continua. These paradoxical reactions highlight the complex immunopathology of pustular psoriasis and underscore the need for individualized therapeutic strategies.

Collamer and Battafarano discovered that palmoplantar pustulosis is more common, followed by plaque psoriasis and guttate psoriasis, with multiple clinical forms potentially existing. Brown and colleagues more frequently described plaque psoriasis, followed by palmoplantar pustulosis [12].

Abbruzzese et al. reported a case of a bioexperienced psoriatic patient (previously treated with etanercept, adalimumab, and golimumab) who developed paradoxical pustular psoriasis after 9 months of secukinumab therapy. The paradoxical eruption improved after treatment with cyclosporine A, contrasting with the patient in case 1 [13].

Tadiotto Cicogna et al. mentioned the case of a 52-year-old woman with psoriatic arthritis undergoing secukinumab therapy for 9 months, who developed a painful eruption with pustules, scaling, and swelling on the fingers of both hands, diagnosed as a paradoxical reaction resembling Hallopeau's acropustulosis (ACH) following anti-IL-17 treatment [14].

Hoshina et al. raised an important issue with a patient who had a documented paradoxical reaction to biologic therapy. The authors could not determine whether the paradoxical reaction was solely due to secukinumab or if other biologic medications, including infliximab or brodalumab, had a partial influence due to the patient's multiple biologic switches [15].

Interestingly, EL-Komy and colleagues described a case in which secukinumab treatment was associated with the onset of psoriasis and pustular eruptions in a 46-year-old woman. Due to financial constraints, the patient had to stop anti-IL-17 therapy for 7 months. Upon reintroduction of secukinumab, psoriasis lesions began to reappear, with plaques on the lower limbs and pustular lesions on the surface. Unlike our patient (case 1 [10]), the author increased the dose of secukinumab and achieved remission of the skin lesions [16].

In the treatment of pustular psoriasis, IL-17 and IL-23 inhibitors are used in some countries. Avallone and colleagues mentioned a better, but inconsistent and statistically nonsignificant, response in patients with pustular psoriasis treated with IL-17 inhibitors compared to IL-23 inhibitors in a retrospective cohort study [17]. Tocilizumab, an anti-IL-6 molecule, may be a therapeutic option for palmoplantar pustular lesions induced by TNF-α treatments, such as infliximab. However, considering the potential for paradoxical psoriasis lesions in patients with psoriatic arthritis, tocilizumab is a limited therapeutic option. IL-6 is involved in the pathogenesis of psoriasis, but the "main players" are TNF-α, IL-17, and IL-23 cytokines [18].

McFeely et al. reported the case of a 45-year-old woman with vulgar psoriasis for 22 years who, after being treated with risankizumab, developed pustular psoriasis on 60% of her body surface [9].

Although multiple cases of paradoxical reactions to ixekizumab have been reported [19–21], there have been no reports of paradoxical reactions to the citrate-free formulation of ixekizumab. This is the first time we mention this occurrence.

Author details

Mihaela Georgescu[1]*, Maria Magdalena Constantin[2], Mădălina Mariana Motoacă[3] and Daniel O. Costache[4]

1 Faculty of Biology, ICUB—SVMP, University of Bucharest, Romania

2 Dermatology Department Colentina Clinical Hospital, University of Medicine and Pharmacy Carol Davila, Romania

3 Dermatology Clinic, Central Military Universitary Emergency Hospital "Carol Davila", Romania

4 Dermatology Discipline, Faculty of Medicine, Carol Davila University of Medicine and Pharmacy, Romania

*Address all correspondence to: georgescucmihaela@gmail.com

References

[1] Baeten D, Kruithof E, Van, Den V, Herssens A, Mielants H, et al. Systematic safety follow up in a cohort of 107 patients with spondyloarthropathy treated with infliximab: A new perspective on the role of host defence in the pathogenesis of the disease? Annals of the Rheumatic Diseases. 2003;**62**(9):829-834

[2] Sfikakis PP, Iliopoulos A, Elezoglou A, Kittas C, Stratigos A. Psoriasis induced by anti-tumor necrosis factor therapy: A paradoxical adverse reaction. Arthritis and Rheumatism. 2005;**52**(8):2513-2518

[3] Mylonas A, Conrad C. Psoriasis: Classical vs. paradoxical. The yin-Yang of TNF and type I interferon. Frontiers in Immunology. 2018;**9**:274

[4] Murphy MJ, Cohen JM, Vesely MD, Damsky W. Paradoxical eruptions to targeted therapies in dermatology: A systematic review and analysis. Journal of the American Academy of Dermatology. 2022;**86**(5):1080-1091

[5] Chokshi A, Demory Beckler M, Laloo A, Kesselman MM. Paradoxical tumor necrosis factor-alpha (TNF-α) inhibitor-induced psoriasis: A systematic review of pathogenesis, clinical presentation, and treatment. Cureus. 2023;**15**(8):e42791

[6] Puig L. Paradoxical reactions: Anti-tumor necrosis factor alpha agents, Ustekinumab, Secukinumab, Ixekizumab, and others. Current Problems in Dermatology. 2018;**53**:49-63

[7] Jiraskova Zakostelska Z, Reiss Z, Tlaskalova-Hogenova H, Rob F. Paradoxical reactions to anti-TNFα and anti-IL-17 treatment in psoriasis patients: Are skin and/or gut microbiota involved? Dermatology and Therapy (Heidelb). 2023;**13**(4):911-933

[8] Nidegger A, Mylonas A, Conrad C. Psoriasis paradoxal induit par anti-TNF—Un challenge en clinique [paradoxical psoriasis induced by anti-TNF—A clinical challenge]. Revue Médicale Suisse. 2019;**15**(644):668-671

[9] McFeely O, Pender E, Victory L, Almutlaq H, Storan E. Risankizumab-induced paradoxical pustular psoriasis. Clinical and Experimental Dermatology. 2022;**47**(3):616-617

[10] Anghel D, Georgescu M, Poenaru M, Orleanu D, Tiplica G. Paradoxical pustular psoriasis in a patient with spondyloarthritis treated with secukinumab. JEADV Clinical Practice. 2023;**2**:951-954

[11] Sin-Soler M, Romaní J, Gamissans M, Riera-Martí N, Lara A, Ribera M. Efectos adversos cutáneos inmunomediados por los anti-TNF: revisión de 30 casos. Actas Dermo-Sifiliográficas. 2024;**115**(1):21-27

[12] Munera-Campos M, Ballesca F, Carrascosa JM. Reacciones paradójicas de los tratamientos biológicos utilizados en psoriasis: revisión de la literatura. Actas Dermo-Sifiliográficas. 2018;**109**(9):791-800

[13] Abbruzzese A, Venerito V, Lopalco G, Fornaro M, Giannotta M, Iannone F. Paradoxical pustular psoriasis in a patient with psoriatic arthritis on secukinumab treatment. Journal of Clinical Rheumatology. 2020;**26**(6):e208-e209

[14] Tadiotto Cicogna G, Messina F, Nalotto L, Szekely S, Alaibac M. Case report: Paradoxical acrodermatitis of Hallopeau-like eruption following

anti-IL-17 therapy. F1000Research. 26 Mar 2019;**8**:336

[15] Hoshina D, Haga N, Furuya K, Sakai M. Paradoxical localized exacerbation of psoriatic eruptions triggered by secukinumab. Clinical and Experimental Dermatology. Aug 2018;**43**(6):718-719

[16] El-Komy M, Amer M, Mostafa A, ElKalioby M. Secukinumab retreatment associated psoriasis flare with pustules. Journal of Dermatological Treatment. 2022;**33**(2):1107-1110

[17] Avallone G, Maronese CA, Murgia G, Carrera CG, Mastorino L, Roccuzzo G, et al. Interleukin-17 vs. interleukin-23 inhibitors in pustular and erythrodermic psoriasis: A retrospective, multicentre cohort study. Journal of Clinical Medicine. 2023;**12**(4):1662

[18] Miceli A, Schmieder GJ. Palmoplantar Psoriasis [Internet]. Treasure Island (FL): StatPearls Publishing; 2022. Available from: https://www ncbi.nlm.nih.gov/books/NBK448142/#_NBK448142_pubdet

[19] Pirro F, Caldarola G, De Simone C, Moretta G, Giovanardi G, Peris K. Multiple paradoxical reactions during ixekizumab therapy. Dermatologic Therapy. 2019;**32**(3):e152

[20] Martínez-Doménech Á, García-Legaz-Martínez M, Magdaleno-Tapial J, Giácaman M, Hernández-Bel P, Pérez-Ferriols A. Paradoxical reversed plantar involvement during ixekizumab therapy for psoriasis. Dermatology Online Journal. 2019;**25**(4):13030/qt4624n3hj

[21] Hlaca N, Zagar T, Kastelan M, Brajac I, Prpic-Massari L. Ixekizumab-induced paradoxical pustular reaction successfully treated with guselkumab. Clinical and Experimental Dermatology. 2021;**46**(8):1572-1573

Chapter 5

Safety Profiles of Biologic Drugs in Psoriasis and Psoriatic Arthritis

Mustafa Ekici

Abstract

Biologic agents have revolutionized the treatment of psoriasis and psoriatic arthritis (PsA) by offering targeted and effective immunomodulation with relatively favorable safety profiles. This chapter provides a comprehensive review of the safety profiles of biologic and targeted synthetic disease-modifying antirheumatic drugs (DMARDs), including TNF-α, IL-17, IL-12/23, and IL-23 inhibitors, and Janus kinase (JAK) and PDE-4 inhibitors. Although TNF-α inhibitors have demonstrated substantial efficacy, they are associated with an increased risk of serious infections, tuberculosis, hepatitis B reactivation, demyelinating disorders, and autoimmune complications. IL-17 and IL-23 inhibitors exhibit a more favorable safety profile, particularly in relation to infection and malignancy, although concerns remain regarding mucocutaneous candidiasis and cardiovascular events. JAK inhibitors are associated with an elevated risk of herpes zoster, thromboembolism, and major adverse cardiovascular events, particularly in older patients and those with preexisting risk factors. Apremilast, a PDE-4 inhibitor, has a low incidence of serious infections and malignancies but may be associated with psychiatric adverse effects, including depression and suicidal ideation. Considerations during pregnancy, breastfeeding, and in the presence of latent infections are also discussed, with an emphasis on screening and prophylactic measures. This chapter underscores the necessity of individualized risk assessment and vigilant monitoring when prescribing advanced therapies for psoriatic disease, ensuring optimized safety while maintaining the therapeutic efficacy of the treatment.

Keywords: psoriasis, psoriatic arthritis, biologic DMARDs, safety profile, targeted synthetic DMARDs

1. Introduction

Biological drugs are modern therapeutic agents used in the treatment of psoriasis and psoriatic arthritis (PsA). These agents are derived from living organisms or produced through genetic engineering, and they specifically target the immune pathways involved in the pathogenesis of the disease. Compared to conventional treatments, biological drugs offer a higher efficacy and a more favorable safety profile. By selectively inhibiting specific cells or molecules that contribute to disease development, they provide a more targeted and effective treatment approach [1]. While the approval status of biologic agents differs from country to country, those frequently

Drug class	Mechanism/target	Approved agents	Indications
TNF-α inhibitors	Block TNF-α	Adalimumab, etanercept, infliximab, golimumab, and certolizumab pegol	Psoriasis, PsA
IL-12/23 (p40) inhibitors	Block IL-12 and IL-23	Ustekinumab	Psoriasis, PsA
IL-23 (p19) inhibitors	Block IL-23	Guselkumab, tildrakizumab, and risankizumab	Psoriasis; guselkumab and risankizumab also for PsA
IL-17 inhibitors	Block IL-17A, IL-17F, or IL-17 receptor	Secukinumab, ixekizumab, brodalumab, and bimekizumab	Psoriasis, PsA
T-cell costimulation inhibitors	Block CD80/86 costimulation	Abatacept	PsA only
Targeted synthetic DMARDs	Inhibit JAKs or PDE-4	Apremilast (PDE4), tofacitinib (JAK1/3), upadacitinib (JAK1), deucravacitinib (TYK2), and baricitinib (JAK1/2)	Psoriasis, PsA

Table 1.
Approved biologic and targeted synthetic DMARDs for Psoriasis & PsA (June 2025) [3, 4].

employed in psoriasis treatment are typically categorized into three primary groups: tumor necrosis factor TNF-α inhibitors, interleukin IL-23 inhibitors, and interleukin IL-17 inhibitors. Although not classified as biological agents, the targeted mechanisms of action of certain synthetic drug classes (targeted synthetic DMARDs), especially in PsA, have led to their consideration as emerging treatment options [2]. Biologic and targeted synthetic disease-modifying antirheumatic drugs (DMARDs) approved for the treatment of psoriasis and PsA by the Food and Drug Administration (FDA) and the European Medicines Agency (EMA) are presented in **Table 1**.

It is well-established that, in addition to their groundbreaking efficacy in the treatment of psoriasis and psoriatic arthritis, both biologic DMARDs (bDMARDs) and targeted synthetic DMARDs (tsDMARDs) are associated with adverse effects that require close monitoring in both randomized controlled trials and real-world clinical practice.

2. TNF-α inhibitors

Tumor necrosis factor-alpha (TNF-α) inhibitors target the cytokine TNF-α, which plays a pivotal role in the immune system and serves as a key mediator in the initiation of inflammation. TNF-α binds to its receptors on the cell surface, thereby triggering an inflammatory response and contributing centrally to the pathogenesis of chronic inflammatory disorders such as rheumatoid arthritis, psoriatic arthritis, and psoriasis. TNF-α inhibitors exert their therapeutic effects through several complementary mechanisms targeting the inflammatory cascade. Primarily, they neutralize TNF-α by binding directly to the molecule, thereby preventing its interaction with cell surface receptors (TNFR1 and TNFR2) and inhibiting subsequent downstream proinflammatory signaling pathways. Furthermore, by neutralizing TNF-α, these agents also reduce the production of other proinflammatory cytokines, like IL-1 and IL-6, whose expression is often TNF-α-dependent, thus limiting the amplification of the inflammatory loop. Finally, by preventing TNF-α–mediated activation of immune cells, these inhibitors mitigate tissue destruction and joint damage, effectively attenuating the progression of structural damage in inflammatory diseases [5, 6].

Adalimumab, infliximab, and golimumab are IgG1 subclass monoclonal antibodies that target the proinflammatory cytokine TNF-α. Although they share a common target, they differ in their molecular structure: adalimumab and golimumab are fully human, whereas infliximab is a chimeric antibody composed of murine variable and human constant regions. Despite these structural differences, all three agents operate via a shared primary mechanism, binding with high affinity to both soluble and membrane-bound TNF-α to block its interaction with its receptors and inhibit downstream signaling. Furthermore, as IgG1 antibodies, they may also induce apoptosis in TNF-α–expressing cells through CDC and antibody-dependent cellular cytotoxicity (ADCC). This multifaceted inhibition of the TNF-α pathway allows these agents to effectively control inflammation and mitigate disease-related structural damage [7]. Structurally distinct from conventional monoclonal antibodies, certolizumab pegol is a PEGylated, humanized antigen-binding fragment (Fab') of an anti-TNF-α antibody. It neutralizes both soluble and membrane-bound TNF-α by preventing interaction with their receptors. Crucially, lacking an Fc region, it does not mediate complement-dependent (CDC) or antibody-dependent cellular cytotoxicity (ADCC). The PEGylation moiety enhances its pharmacokinetic profile, prolonging its half-life and duration of action [8]. Etanercept, in contrast, is a dimeric fusion protein comprising the extracellular ligand-binding domain of human TNF receptor 2 (TNFR2) fused to the Fc portion of human IgG1. This structure allows it to bind and neutralize not only TNF-α but also TNF-α (lymphotoxin). While its Fc region enables CDC and ADCC, these effector functions are generally considered weaker than those of anti-TNF monoclonal antibodies. Through this dual neutralization mechanism, etanercept effectively attenuates the downstream inflammatory cascade [7].

2.1 Safety profiles of anti-TNF drugs

While anti-TNF agents have transformed the management of chronic inflammatory diseases, their use is associated with significant safety considerations that demand careful risk-benefit assessment. Common adverse effects include a spectrum of gastrointestinal and behavioral symptoms. More rarely, patients may experience systemic symptoms such as fatigue, myalgia, nausea, and anorexia, which typically resolve upon discontinuation of the therapy. The most prominent risk is an increased susceptibility to serious infections, including the reactivation of latent tuberculosis and hepatitis B. Furthermore, long-term therapy has been linked to a potential increase in certain malignancies and the emergence of autoimmune phenomena. These risks necessitate comprehensive pretreatment screening, vigilant patient monitoring, and an individualized approach to ensure therapeutic safety.

2.1.1 Infection

TNF-alpha plays a pivotal role in host defense against various pathogens; consequently, its therapeutic inhibition is associated with an increased risk of serious infections.

According to the most comprehensive meta-analysis to date as of 2024, which included 61 randomized controlled trials and 20,458 patients with rheumatoid arthritis (RA), PsA, and ankylosing spondylitis (AS), TNF-α inhibitors are associated with varying degrees of infection risk. Certolizumab pegol was found to significantly increase the risk of serious infections compared to placebo (OR: 2.28, 95% CI: 1.13–4.62), as well as compared to golimumab (OR: 2.67, 95% CI: 1.14–6.26) and etanercept (OR: 2.41, 95% CI: 1.14–5.08). Adalimumab (OR: 1.27, 95% CI: 0.85–1.88), infliximab (OR: 1.39, 95% CI: 0.72–2.68), and golimumab (OR: 0.69, 95% CI: 0.36–1.35) did not show statistically significant increases in serious infection risk when compared to placebo. The cumulative ranking for serious infections placed certolizumab pegol as the highest-risk agent (90.7%), followed by infliximab (73.1%) and adalimumab (69.5%), while etanercept (17.0%) and golimumab (12.8%) had the lowest rankings [9].

For the outcome of any infection, both certolizumab pegol (OR: 1.40, 95% CI: 1.11–1.76) and adalimumab (OR: 1.18, 95% CI: 1.06–1.30) showed significantly elevated risks compared to placebo. No significant associations were observed between TNF inhibitors and the risk of opportunistic infections ($p > 0.05$) or herpes zoster (OR: 1.50, 95% CI: 0.72–3.11); however, TNF inhibitors did significantly increase the risk of tuberculosis (OR: 2.21, 95% CI: 1.05–4.66). These findings suggest that while TNF inhibitors are effective treatments for inflammatory arthritis, agents such as etanercept and golimumab may present a more favorable safety profile regarding infection risk, particularly in patients with higher baseline vulnerability [9].

The American College of Rheumatology (ACR) guidelines contraindicate the use of TNF-α inhibitors in patients with various active or untreated infections. These include active bacterial infections, herpes zoster, invasive fungal infections, non-healing skin ulcers, and active or untreated tuberculosis. Furthermore, their use is contraindicated in acute or untreated chronic hepatitis B, as well as in patients with chronic hepatitis B or C who have significant liver dysfunction (Child-Pugh class B or C), given the heightened risk of severe complications under immunosuppression [10].

Treatment with anti-TNF agents carries a significant risk of hepatitis B virus (HBV) reactivation, particularly in patients with chronic HBV infection. Therefore, comprehensive HBV screening (HBsAg, anti-HBc, anti-HBs) is essential prior to initiating therapy. Prophylactic antiviral treatment—preferably with low-resistance agents such as entecavir or tenofovir—is strongly recommended in HBsAg-positive individuals, including inactive carriers with low HBV DNA levels, as it significantly reduces the risk of reactivation and liver injury. In contrast, patients with resolved HBV infection (HBsAg negative, anti-HBc-positive) generally do not require prophylaxis, although close monitoring of ALT and HBV DNA is advised. Antiviral prophylaxis may be considered in select high-risk cases, such as those with negative anti-HBs or additional immunosuppressive therapy. Prompt initiation of antiviral treatment is critical upon signs of reactivation [11].

Patients receiving anti-TNF therapy face a significantly increased risk of developing tuberculosis (TB) compared to the general population. The incidence rate exhibits substantial geographic variation, with reported global estimates around 9 to 10 cases per 1000 patients. Rates are highest in Asia (13.47 per 1000) and South America (11.75 per 1000) and considerably lower in Europe (6.28 per 1000) and North America (4.34 per 1000). Consistent with these regional trends, a large Turkish cohort of over 10,000 patients reported a TB incidence of 0.69%, equivalent to approximately 7 cases per 1000 patients [12, 13]. Anti-TNF-α agents confer a greater risk of TB compared to biologic therapies with other mechanisms of action. Furthermore, a clear risk differential exists within the anti-TNF class itself: monoclonal antibody-based agents (infliximab, adalimumab, golimumab, and certolizumab) are associated with a higher incidence of TB than the soluble TNF-α receptor fusion protein, etanercept [14]. Therefore, comprehensive screening for both active and latent TB is mandatory prior to initiating anti-TNF therapy. This screening protocol involves three core components: a thorough medical history focusing on TB exposure and risk factors, a posteroanterior chest X-ray to exclude active disease, and testing for latent TB infection (LTBI). For LTBI screening, either the tuberculin skin test (TST) or an interferon-gamma release assay (IGRA) is acceptable, though IGRA is generally preferred due to its higher specificity [15, 16]. In latent tuberculosis screening, if the tuberculin skin test (TST/PPD) is used as the initial test, an induration of ≥5 mm is considered positive and should prompt initiation of prophylactic treatment. In cases with induration <5 mm, IGRA testing or a repeat PPD (booster) after 1–3 weeks is recommended. If the repeated test is positive, latent tuberculosis prophylaxis should be initiated [17].

2.1.2 Malignancy

Psoriasis is strongly associated with a range of comorbidities, including depression, metabolic syndrome, and atherosclerotic cardiovascular disease. An increased risk of certain malignancies—such as lymphoma, nonmelanoma skin cancer (NMSC), and lung cancer—is also well-documented, an association potentially driven by shared lifestyle risk factors like smoking and obesity. Compounding this intrinsic risk, some psoriasis treatments, including phototherapy and systemic immunosuppressants, have themselves raised concerns about malignancy, though the evidence remains equivocal. According to the most recent comprehensive meta-analysis, among patients with psoriasis or psoriatic arthritis treated with TNF-α inhibitors, a significantly increased risk was found only for nonmelanoma skin cancer in those with psoriatic arthritis (two studies; SIR 1.839; 95% CI: 1.160–2.916; $P = 0.010$) and for squamous cell carcinoma overall (three studies; SIR 2.839; 95% CI: 1.642–4.909; $P < 0.001$). Other cancer types showed no significant increase [18, 19].

2.1.3 Demyelinating disease

The use of anti-TNF agents has been linked to an increased risk of demyelinating disorders affecting both the central and peripheral nervous systems. These rare but serious complications—such as multiple sclerosis-like syndromes, optic neuritis, and transverse myelitis—typically emerge within the first 2 years of therapy.

A comprehensive meta-analysis by Wenhui Xie et al. quantified this risk, demonstrating a significantly higher incidence of inflammatory CNS events with TNF-α inhibitors compared to conventional therapies (RR 1.36). Notably, this elevated risk was not observed when TNF-α inhibitors were compared with other biologics or Janus kinase inhibitors. Subgroup analyses showed no significant variation in risk across underlying autoimmune diseases. However, within the anti-TNF class, certolizumab pegol was uniquely associated with a significantly increased risk (RR 1.39), while other monoclonal antibodies and etanercept showed comparable safety profiles [20]. Given the potential risk, anti-TNF-α agents are typically avoided in patients with known demyelinating disorders, such as multiple sclerosis. If signs suggestive of demyelination emerge during treatment, discontinuation of therapy is generally recommended. Additionally, some clinicians proceed with caution when prescribing TNF-α inhibitors to patients with a family history of multiple sclerosis.

2.1.4 Cardiovascular disease

Patients with psoriatic arthritis have a 43% higher risk of cardiovascular diseases—with myocardial infarction and heart failure risks increased by 68 and 31%, respectively—and those with severe psoriasis show a 70% higher risk of myocardial infarction and a 37% increase in cardiovascular mortality, according to a recent meta-analysis of observational studies comparing outcomes with the general population [21, 22]. In patients with psoriasis and psoriatic arthritis, anti-TNF agents such as adalimumab, etanercept, and infliximab are generally considered cardioprotective, with large cohort studies and meta-analyses demonstrating significantly reduced risks of major adverse cardiovascular events (MACE), myocardial infarction, stroke, and heart failure compared to conventional systemic or topical therapies (e.g., HR 0.74; IRR 0.77), though caution is warranted in individuals with preexisting heart failure, as some reports suggest a potential—albeit low—risk of new or worsening heart failure, particularly when compared to ustekinumab (HR 0.64 in favor of ustekinumab) [23, 24]. The use of targeted TNF-α inhibitors may contribute to the onset or worsening of heart failure. In patients with symptomatic heart failure, alternative treatment options should be considered. If heart failure develops during TNF-α inhibitor therapy, a drug-induced etiology should be suspected, and the medication should be discontinued.

Although anti-TNF agents are generally associated with reduced cardiovascular risk in psoriatic disease, recent findings suggest a more complex picture. A large network meta-analysis (40 studies; 126,961 patients with rheumatoid arthritis, ankylosing spondylitis, psoriatic arthritis, and inflammatory bowel disease) demonstrated an increased risk of MACE compared to placebo for several advanced therapies. Specifically, elevated risks were observed with anti-TNF-α agents (OR 2.49; 95% CrI, 1.14–5.62), JAK inhibitors (OR 2.64; 95% CrI, 1.26–5.99), and IL-12/23 inhibitors (OR 3.15; 95% CrI, 1.01–13.35). Notably, the magnitude of risk was similar across these drug classes and consistent regardless of the underlying disease, highlighting the need for long-term safety data as biologic use continues [25].

2.1.5 Autoimmunity and autoantibodies

Anti-TNF agents used in psoriatic arthritis and psoriasis carry certain risks related to autoimmunity and antidrug antibody (ADA) formation. Recent comprehensive meta-analyses have shown that during anti-TNF therapy, the incidence of ADA development can reach 29.7% for infliximab and 31.8% for adalimumab, whereas it remains substantially lower for etanercept at 2.2%. The presence of ADAs may reduce therapeutic efficacy and increase the risk of injection-site reactions; however, concomitant use of immunosuppressants such as methotrexate may help mitigate ADA formation [26].

Anti-TNF therapy has been associated with the induction of various autoantibodies, most commonly antinuclear antibodies (ANA), followed by anti-double-stranded DNA (anti-dsDNA) and antiphospholipid antibodies. Reported frequencies vary widely depending on the specific agent, underlying disease, and concomitant immunosuppressive treatments. In clinical studies, ANA positivity was observed in 29–77% of patients treated with infliximab, 11–36% with etanercept, and 13% with adalimumab, while anti-dsDNA antibodies were detected in 10–29%, 5–15%, and 5% of these patients, respectively. Although the presence of autoantibodies is often clinically silent, they may precede or accompany drug-induced autoimmune syndromes. Notably, in patients with psoriasis receiving TNF inhibitors, an increased frequency of antiphospholipid antibodies has been reported, although no clinical features of antiphospholipid syndrome (APS) were observed. The most commonly reported autoimmune conditions include lupus-like syndrome, cutaneous or systemic vasculitis, antiphospholipid syndrome, and sarcoidosis. More rarely, inflammatory myopathies (e.g., dermatomyositis, polymyositis), uveitis, autoimmune hepatitis, and interstitial lung disease have been observed. These manifestations are generally reversible upon discontinuation of the TNF inhibitor, but in some cases, additional immunosuppressive therapy is required. Therefore, clinicians should monitor for signs of autoimmune activation, particularly in patients with a personal or familial predisposition to autoimmunity [27].

2.1.6 Pregnancy and breastfeeding

One of the primary concerns regarding the use of biologic agents during pregnancy is the potential risk of teratogenicity during organogenesis (weeks 3–8) and postnatal immunosuppression in the newborn. Although transplacental antibody transfer is thought to begin around the 13th week of gestation, most of the transfer occurs during the third trimester, particularly after week 28, and increases progressively until delivery. Placental IgG transfer is mediated by an active transcytosis mechanism through syncytiotrophoblasts, involving binding of the Fc portion of IgG antibodies to the neonatal Fc receptor (FcRn). Among the IgG subclasses, IgG1 is transferred most efficiently, whereas IgG2 and IgG3 exhibit markedly lower transfer rates owing to their reduced affinity for FcRn. Consequently, monoclonal antibodies of the IgG1 subclass, such as TNF inhibitors, can cross the placenta in significant amounts during late pregnancy, whereas agents such as certolizumab pegol, which lack an Fc region, are not actively transported and thus demonstrate minimal to no placental transfer [28]. For women with well-controlled disease using TNF inhibitors known to cross the placenta, such as infliximab, adalimumab, and golimumab, there is generally no need to switch to certolizumab pegol before or during pregnancy. Certolizumab pegol is considered safe throughout all trimesters because of its minimal placental transfer and does not necessitate any modification to the infant vaccination schedule. In patients with a low risk of disease flare, treatment discontinuation may be considered at gestational week 20 for infliximab, week 28 for adalimumab and golimumab, and week 32 for etanercept, allowing standard live vaccinations, including rotavirus, to begin at 8 weeks of age. However, if disease activity requires the continuation of therapy during pregnancy, live vaccines should be delayed until 6 months of age. Resumption of TNF inhibitor therapy in the postpartum period can occur as early as possible, regardless of breastfeeding status, provided that there are no infectious or surgical complications. All TNF inhibitors are considered compatible with breastfeeding [29].

3. IL-17, IL-12/23, and IL-23 inhibitors

Anti-IL-17 agents exert their effects by targeting proinflammatory cytokines, particularly IL-17A and IL-17F. IL-17A is primarily produced by Th17 cells, but also by $CD8^{+}$ T cells, $\gamma\delta$ T cells, and natural killer T cells. These cytokines play a key role in host defense by promoting neutrophil recruitment to sites of inflammation, stimulating epithelial cells to release antimicrobial peptides and chemokines, and enhancing barrier integrity. However, excessive and dysregulated IL-17 production contributes to chronic inflammation and tissue damage in autoimmune diseases, such as psoriasis and psoriatic arthritis. Anti-IL-17 therapies, such as secukinumab and ixekizumab, which neutralize IL-17A; bimekizumab, which neutralizes IL-17 A-F; and brodalumab, which blocks the IL-17A receptor (IL-17RA), suppress these pathogenic responses by preventing the accumulation of inflammatory cells and mediators in target tissues, such as the skin and joints. Compared to TNF inhibitors, anti-IL-17 agents have a more localized immunomodulatory effect, resulting in a more modest increase in the risk of infection [30].

IL-12 and IL-23 are proinflammatory cytokines involved in immune-mediated inflammation and share a common p40 subunit; IL-12 also contains a p35 subunit, whereas IL-23 includes a p19 subunit. Ustekinumab is a monoclonal antibody that targets the shared p40 subunit, thereby inhibiting both IL-12–mediated Th1 and IL-23–mediated Th17 responses. In contrast, next-generation IL-23 inhibitors, such as guselkumab, risankizumab, tildrakizumab, and mirikizumab, selectively bind to the p19 subunit, specifically blocking IL-23 activity. By preventing IL-23–induced activation of Th17 cells and the subsequent production of proinflammatory cytokines such as IL-17, these agents reduce inflammation more precisely, with potentially improved safety and efficacy profiles [31].

3.1 Safety profiles of IL-17, IL-12/23, and IL-23 inhibitors

3.1.1 Infection

IL-17 plays a critical role in mucocutaneous immunity, particularly in host defense against fungal pathogens, such as Candida species. Consequently, treatment with anti-IL-17 agents is associated with a markedly increased risk of oropharyngeal, esophageal, and cutaneous candidiasis. Real-world data and clinical trials suggest a 2- to 40-fold increase in the risk of candidiasis among patients receiving anti-IL-17 therapy, with oral and esophageal infections being the most frequently reported. These infections are typically mild and manageable with antifungal therapy; however, long-term treatment warrants careful monitoring. Additionally, upper respiratory tract infections (e.g., nasopharyngitis) and urinary tract infections have been reported more commonly in patients receiving anti-IL-17 agents than in those receiving placebo, although the overall risk of serious infection remains low. Importantly, anti-IL-17 therapy does not significantly increase the risk of herpes zoster [30, 32, 33]. Anti-IL-12/23 agents and selective anti-IL-23 inhibitors are generally considered safe with respect to infection risk and have not been associated with a significant increase in the incidence of serious infections. Large meta-analyses and real-world data suggest a slight increase in upper respiratory tract infections, particularly nasopharyngitis, but no meaningful elevation in the incidence of lower respiratory tract infections, viral illnesses, serious bacterial infections, or invasive fungal infections. The rate of serious infections in patients treated with these agents is approximately 2.4%, comparable to that observed with anti-NF. Notably, no cases of deep or invasive fungal infections have been reported, and the risk of superficial candidiasis appears to be substantially lower than that associated with anti-IL-17 therapy [34].

The risk of hepatitis B virus (HBV) reactivation associated with anti-IL-17, anti-IL-12/23, and anti-IL-23 inhibitors is generally low but varies according to the patient's HBV status. In patients with chronic HBV infection (defined by positive HBsAg or detectable HBV DNA), the overall reactivation risk during treatment with these biologics is <6%, with reported rates of 4% for anti-IL-17 agents and 2% and 0% for anti-IL-12/23 and anti-IL-23 agents, respectively. However, in chronically infected individuals not receiving antiviral prophylaxis, reactivation rates may reach 28%. In contrast, the risk of reactivation in patients with previous HBV infection (HBcAb positive, HBsAg negative) is much lower and is estimated to be approximately 4.7%. No significant differences in reactivation rates were observed among the different biological classes. Therefore, antiviral prophylaxis is recommended for patients with chronic HBV infection undergoing treatment with these agents, whereas close monitoring may be sufficient for those with a history of HBV exposure [35].

Compared to TNF inhibitors, anti-IL-17, anti-IL-12/23, and anti-IL-23 agents are considered substantially safer with respect to the risk of TB reactivation. Large observational studies, meta-analyses, and real-world data have demonstrated TB reactivation rates of less than 1% in patients with LTBI treated with anti-IL-17 and anti-IL-23 inhibitors, reported at approximately 0.78 and 0.17%, respectively. Although data on anti-IL-12/23 agents are limited, no significant TB reactivation has been documented to date. Nevertheless, screening for LTBI is recommended prior to initiating therapy, particularly in TB-endemic regions. While chemoprophylaxis may be considered in LTBI-positive patients, the decision can be approached more flexibly than with TNF inhibitors, given the lower risk of reactivation [36].

3.1.2 Malignancy

The malignancy risk profiles of anti-IL-17, anti-IL-12/23, and anti-IL-23 inhibitors are generally considered favorable. Comprehensive meta-analyses and long-term observational studies have shown no significant increase in the overall cancer risk with either short- or long-term use of these agents. For example, the short-term malignancy risk ratio was reported as 0.83 (95% CI: 0.41–1.71) for anti-IL-17 inhibitors and 0.87 (95% CI: 0.37–2.04) for anti-IL-23 inhibitors. Longitudinal data also indicate that the incidence of nonmelanoma skin cancer and other malignancies is comparable to or lower than that in the general population. Similarly, studies on anti-IL-12/23 inhibitors suggest no meaningful increase in cancer risk with long-term use, and the risk appears to be similar to or lower than that associated with TNF inhibitors. Importantly, no significant increase in the incidence of melanoma or nonmelanoma skin cancer has been observed with any of these agents [37–39].

3.1.3 Cardiovascular disease

Recent evidence has raised concerns regarding the cardiovascular safety of various biologic and targeted synthetic therapies used in immune-mediated inflammatory diseases (IMIDs), including PsA, rheumatoid arthritis, inflammatory bowel disease, and ankylosing spondylitis. A comprehensive network meta-analysis of 40 studies encompassing 126,961 patients found that anti-TNF-α agents (OR 2.49; 95% CrI 1.14–5.62), JAK inhibitors (OR 2.64; 95% CrI 1.26–5.99), and anti-IL-12/23 agents (OR 3.15; 95% CrI 1.01–13.35) were each associated with an increased risk of major adverse cardiovascular events (MACE) compared with placebo, irrespective of the underlying disease type. Complementing these findings, a large nationwide cohort study of 11,395 PsA patients in France, excluding those with prior cardiovascular disease, reported a significantly higher MACE risk for new users of IL-12/23 (HR 2.0; 95% CI 1.3–3.0) and IL-17 inhibitors (HR 1.9; 95% CI 1.2–3.0) compared with TNF inhibitors, while apremilast showed no significant increase (HR 1.3; 95% CI 0.8–2.2).

Together, these data suggest that although the absolute number of cardiovascular events remains low, certain biologic classes—particularly IL-12/23 and IL-17 inhibitors—may carry a higher relative cardiovascular risk than TNF inhibitors in patients with PsA and related IMIDs, warranting further prospective investigation [25, 40].

3.1.4 Pregnancy and breastfeeding

Current recommendations suggest that interleukin-17 (IL-17) and interleukin-12/23 (IL-12/23) inhibitors should be discontinued at conception due to limited data on teratogenicity, although available evidence does not indicate harm from in utero exposure. In cases where no safer alternatives exist, these agents may be considered for the management of severe maternal disease during pregnancy. If IL-17 inhibitors or IL-12/23 inhibitors are used in the third trimester, it is recommended to delay all live vaccinations in infants until they are 6 months of age. Although the evidence remains limited, both IL-17 and IL-12/23 inhibitors are considered compatible with breastfeeding [29].

4. JAK inhibitors

Janus kinase (JAK) inhibitors target the JAK family of intracellular tyrosine kinases, which play critical roles in cytokine and growth factor signaling. The JAK family consists of four members: JAK1, JAK2, JAK3, and TYK2. These kinases are associated with receptors for various cytokines, including interleukins and interferons. Upon ligand-binding, receptor-associated JAKs become activated and phosphorylate the receptor, which in turn leads to the phosphorylation and nuclear translocation of signal transducer and transcription activator (STAT) proteins, initiating the transcription of target genes. By blocking this signaling cascade, JAK inhibitors suppress multiple proinflammatory and immune-mediated pathways, thereby reducing inflammation and immune activation. Different JAK inhibitors exhibit varying selectivity for specific JAK isoforms: tofacitinib primarily targets JAK1 and JAK3, baricitinib inhibits JAK1 and JAK2, and upadacitinib is more selective for JAK1 [41].

4.1 Safety profiles of JAK inhibitors

4.1.1 Infection

JAK inhibitors are associated with an increased risk of infection compared to placebo, particularly at higher doses. The most frequently reported infections were upper respiratory tract, urinary tract, and skin infections. Serious infections, such as pneumonia and sepsis, are rare but have been observed more frequently in older patients and those receiving concomitant corticosteroids. This risk appears to be dose-dependent, particularly for tofacitinib, baricitinib, and upadacitinib. Meta-analyses have shown that herpes zoster infections occur two to three times more often in patients receiving JAK inhibitors than in those on placebo (Asians and rheumatoid arthritis patients have a greater prevalence), with most cases being mild to moderate and not requiring treatment discontinuation [42–45].

JAK inhibitors carry a substantial risk of hepatitis B virus (HBV) reactivation in patients with chronic infection (HBsAg-positive), with reported rates ranging from

14–28%, particularly in the absence of antiviral prophylaxis. In contrast, patients with resolved HBV infection (anti-HBc positive, HBsAg negative) have a lower but non-negligible risk, estimated to be between 2 and 5%. The use of prophylactic antiviral therapy, such as entecavir or tenofovir, can reduce reactivation rates in HBsAg-positive individuals to as low as 0–6%. While prophylaxis is generally not recommended for those with resolved infections, close monitoring with serial HBV DNA and liver function tests is essential. The risk of HBV reactivation with JAK inhibitors appears similar to or slightly lower than that observed with TNF inhibitors and other biologics; however, it remains clinically significant in patients with chronic infection, warranting preventive measures. Current guidelines recommend HBV serologic screening (HBsAg, anti-HBc, and anti-HBs) for all patients before initiating JAK inhibitor therapy, initiation of prophylaxis in HBsAg-positive individuals, and regular monitoring in at-risk populations [35, 46].

The risk of TB reactivation with JAK inhibitors is generally lower than that observed with TNF inhibitors and may be comparable to or slightly higher than that observed with IL-17/23 inhibitors. Clinical trials and real-world data indicate that TB reactivation rates remain very low with appropriate screening and prophylaxis. Current guidelines recommend systematic TB screening, including tuberculin skin testing (TST) or interferon-gamma release assay (IGRA) and chest radiography, for all patients prior to initiating JAK inhibitor therapy. In cases of latent TB infection (LTBI), prophylactic treatment with isoniazid or rifampicin should be initiated, and JAK inhibitors may be safely started 1 month after the initiation of prophylaxis. These precautions are essential to minimize the risk of TB reactivation during JAK inhibitor treatment [47, 48].

4.1.2 Malignancy

In large meta-analyses, the overall incidence of malignancy among patients treated with JAK inhibitors was reported to be 1.15–1.26 per 100 patient-years. Compared with placebo (IRR 0.71–0.81) or methotrexate (IRR 0.73–0.77), JAK inhibitors were not associated with a significant increase in the risk of malignancy. However, when compared with TNF inhibitors, the risk appears to be significantly higher (IRR 1.50–1.54). While the incidence of melanoma is similar between JAK inhibitors and biologic agents, nonmelanoma skin cancer (NMSC) rates may be higher with JAK inhibitors, with an incidence rate of approximately 0.45 per 100 patient-years. For solid organ malignancies, including breast, colon, lung, and prostate cancers, no meaningful difference in risk was observed between JAK inhibitors and TNF or IL-17 inhibitors. Importantly, malignancies remained rare across all treatment groups [49, 50].

Before initiating JAK inhibitor therapy, a thorough assessment of personal and family history of malignancy, along with an evaluation of individual risk factors, is recommended. During treatment, regular skin examinations and dermatological evaluations are advised, particularly because of the elevated risk of nonmelanoma skin cancer (NMSC). Standard cancer screening protocols, such as those for breast, colon, and prostate cancer, should be followed based on the patient's age and overall risk profile. For patients receiving long-term therapy, especially those with additional risk factors such as smoking, advanced age, or a history of malignancy, more frequent monitoring is warranted. Regulatory agencies, such as the FDA and EMA, recommend ongoing surveillance of patients treated with JAK inhibitors owing to the potential risk of cancer [51].

4.1.3 Cardiovascular disease

In the general population of patients with psoriasis and psoriatic arthritis, the incidence of MACE associated with JAK inhibitors has been reported to be low, with no significant increase observed compared to placebo or other biologic agents [52]. However, in patients with established cardiovascular risk factors, such as prior cardiovascular disease, advanced age, diabetes, hypertension, dyslipidemia, or metabolic syndrome, the risk of MACE appears to be notably elevated. In the ORAL surveillance trial, tofacitinib was associated with a higher incidence of MACE than TNF inhibitors in patients aged ≥65 years with additional risk factors [53]. JAK inhibitors, particularly tofacitinib and upadacitinib, have also been shown to increase serum LDL and HDL cholesterol levels, although the LDL/HDL ratio typically remains unchanged, and a direct causal link between these lipid changes and MACE risk has not been definitively established [54]. Regulatory agencies such as the EMA and FDA recommend the cautious use of JAK inhibitors in high-risk patients, with regular assessment of cardiovascular risk. In clinical practice, evaluation and monitoring of cardiovascular risk factors should be performed before and during JAK inhibitor therapy, with appropriate management strategies implemented.

The risk of venous thromboembolism (VTE), particularly deep vein thrombosis (DVT) and pulmonary embolism (PE), has emerged as a notable safety concern in patients treated with JAK inhibitors, such as tofacitinib, baricitinib, and upadacitinib. Regulatory agencies, including the FDA and EMA, have issued warnings regarding the thromboembolic risk, particularly in older patients and those with cardiovascular comorbidities. Although large meta-analyses and randomized controlled trials in dermatologic populations (including psoriasis) have not demonstrated a significant increase in DVT or VTE risk (OR 0.52; 95% CI 0.26–1.04), pharmacovigilance data, such as from the FAERS database, have identified higher reporting signals for DVT among patients aged over 65 years, particularly males, treated with tofacitinib and baricitinib, with similar trends observed for upadacitinib. The elevated thromboembolic risk may be more attributable to underlying patient-related factors, such as age, immobility, and comorbidities, rather than a direct drug effect. Therefore, caution is advised when prescribing JAK inhibitors to patients aged >50 years, those with cardiovascular risk factors, a history of thromboembolic events, or prolonged immobility [51, 55, 56].

4.1.4 Pregnancy and breastfeeding

Due to limited data, JAK inhibitors are not recommended for use during pregnancy and should ideally be discontinued at least 2 weeks before planned conception. Similarly, their use during breastfeeding is discouraged, as they are likely to transfer into breastmilk, and the potential effects on the infant remain unknown. Until more robust safety data become available, JAK inhibitors should be avoided during pregnancy and lactation [29].

5. PDE-4 inhibitor

Apremilast is an oral small-molecule inhibitor of phosphodiesterase 4 (PDE-4), which is responsible for degrading intracellular cyclic adenosine monophosphate (cAMP). By elevating cAMP levels, apremilast downregulates the production of key proinflammatory cytokines involved in the pathogenesis of psoriasis and psoriatic arthritis, including TNF-α, IL-23, IL-17A, IL-17F, and IL-22, while upregulating the anti-inflammatory cytokine IL-10. It also promotes the expansion of IL-10–producing regulatory B cells (Bregs) and reduces the number of proinflammatory Th1, Th17, and NKT cells. These combined effects result in the suppression of both cutaneous and joint inflammation, contributing to clinical improvement in psoriatic disease [57, 58].

5.1 Safety profiles of PDE-4 inhibitor

5.1.1 Infection

Comprehensive meta-analyses and phase III randomized controlled trials have shown that apremilast is associated with a slight increase in overall infection rates compared to placebo; however, it does not significantly elevate the risk of serious infections requiring hospitalization or pose a life-threatening threat. The most commonly reported infections are mild and transient, such as upper respiratory tract infections and nasopharyngitis. Notably, the incidence of serious infections with apremilast is comparable to that observed with placebo and other systemic agents. Additionally, the risk of opportunistic infections, including tuberculosis, hepatitis, and herpes zoster, is considered very low, with no cases of TB reactivation or severe viral infections reported in clinical trials [59, 60].

5.1.2 Malignancy

Real-world data and clinical trials consistently indicate that apremilast is associated with a low risk of malignancy in patients with psoriasis and psoriatic arthritis, with no significant increase compared with other systemic therapies. In a large 5-year cohort study, the incidence of hematologic malignancies, nonmelanoma skin cancers, and solid tumors was reported to be either zero or very low among apremilast users. Long-term phase III trials (≥156 weeks) have similarly shown that the rates of malignancy, including hematologic, cutaneous, and solid tumors, remain low and comparable to placebo, with no emerging safety signals over extended follow-up. Importantly, apremilast has also demonstrated a favorable safety profile in patients with a history of cancer, with no reported cases of cancer recurrence or progression during treatment in real-world studies. Given its benign oncologic profile, apremilast is often considered a safer alternative to biologic agents, such as TNF inhibitors, particularly in patients with a history of malignancy or elevated cancer risk [60–62].

5.1.3 Cardiovascular disease

In large cohort and real-world studies, apremilast has been associated with a low risk of MACE, including myocardial infarction, stroke, and revascularization, in patients with psoriasis or psoriatic arthritis. No significant increase in MACE risk was observed compared to that with TNF inhibitors or other biologic agents. Data from the French national health database and the U.S. The MarketScan registry confirmed that apremilast users had low MACE incidence rates, with myocardial infarction and stroke rates reported at 2.5 and 1.6 per 1000 person-years, respectively (HR 1.3; 95% CI 0.8–2.2 vs. TNF inhibitors). Compared with IL-12/23 and IL-17 inhibitors, the cardiovascular safety profile of apremilast appears similar or slightly more favorable. Moreover, apremilast treatment has been linked to modest reductions in body fat mass and slight decreases in blood pressure. Adiposity reduction is positively correlated with improvements in disease activity [40, 63–65].

5.1.4 Psychiatric risk profile of apremilast

Although generally well tolerated, apremilast has been associated with psychiatric adverse events in a small subset of patients with psoriasis. In controlled clinical trials, including ESTEEM, PALACE, LIBERATE, and EMBRACE, mild to moderate psychiatric side effects, including depression and suicidal ideation, were reported infrequently, with depression rates ranging from 0.6 to 2.5% over long-term follow-up. Suicidal ideation occurred in isolated cases, typically in patients with a history of psychiatric disorders. Real-world data from large registries and cohort studies (e.g., MarketScan, APOLO, and national multicenter trials in Europe) have similarly reported low but notable incidences of depression and suicidal thoughts, often resolving after discontinuation of the drug. In one study, the incidence rates of treated anxiety and depression were 9.2 and 4.6 per 1000 person-years, respectively, with an increased frequency of psychiatric events observed in patients receiving concomitant corticosteroids. Following post-marketing surveillance data from over 105,000 patients and the reporting of 65 psychiatric adverse events, including five completed suicides and multiple cases of suicidal ideation, the European Medicines Agency (EMA) issued a safety communication regarding apremilast in October 2016. Subsequent guidelines recommend careful risk-benefit evaluation before initiating or continuing apremilast therapy in patients with a history of psychiatric illness or those using other psychotropic medications. Psychiatric symptoms should be actively monitored during follow-up visits, and the drug should be discontinued if new or worsening depression, suicidal ideation, or suicide attempts occur [66].

Author details

Mustafa Ekici
Department of Rheumatology, Ankara Bilkent City Hospital, Ankara, Türkiye

*Address all correspondence to: ekici42mustafa@gmail.com

References

[1] Weger W. Current status and new developments in the treatment of psoriasis and psoriatic arthritis with biological agents. British Journal of Pharmacology. 2010;**160**(4):810-820

[2] Kamata M, Tada Y. Efficacy and safety of biologics for psoriasis and psoriatic arthritis and their impact on comorbidities: A literature review. International Journal of Molecular Sciences. 2020;**21**(5):1690

[3] Drugs@FDA. FDA-Approved Drugs [Internet]. Available from: https://www.accessdata.fda.gov/scripts/cder/daf/index.cfm [Accessed: June 21, 2025]

[4] Medicines – European Medicines Agency (EMA). 2023 [Internet]. Available from: https://www.ema.europa.eu/en/medicines [Accessed: June 21, 2025]

[5] In JD, Lee AH, Shin HY, Song HR, Park JH, Kang TB, et al. The role of tumor necrosis factor alpha (TNF-α) in autoimmune disease and current TNF-α inhibitors in therapeutics. International Journal of Molecular Sciences. 2021;**22**(5):2719

[6] Leone GM, Mangano K, Petralia MC, Nicoletti F, Fagone P. Past, present and (foreseeable) future of biological anti-TNF alpha therapy. Journal of Clinical Medicine. 2023;**12**(4):1630

[7] Lim H, Lee S, Lee H, Lee J, Son J, Shin W, et al. Structural biology of the TNFα antagonists used in the treatment of rheumatoid arthritis. International Journal of Molecular Sciences. 2018;**19**(3):768

[8] Pasut G. Pegylation of biological molecules and potential benefits: Pharmacological properties of Certolizumab Pegol. BioDrugs. 2014;**28**(S1):15-23

[9] Jiang Z, Zou Y, Li G, Zhao S, Zhang W. Comparisons of infection events associated with tumor necrosis factor inhibitors in patients with inflammatory arthritis: A systematic review and network meta-analysis. Frontiers in Pharmacology. 2024;**15**:1376262

[10] Winthrop KL. Tumor Necrosis Factor-Alpha Inhibitors: Bacterial, Viral, and Fungal Infections. UpToDate. Walth Mass Wolters Kluwer [Internet]; 2014. Available from: https://www.uptodate.com/contents/tumor-necrosis-factor-alpha-inhibitors-bacterial-viral-and-fungal-infections [Accessed: June 22, 2025]

[11] Karadağ Ö, Kaşifoğlu T, Özer B, Kaymakoğlu S, Kuş Y, İnanç M, et al. Guideline of the viral hepatitis screening before biologic agents use in patients with rheumatic diseases. RAED Dergisi. 2015;**7**(1):28-32

[12] Kisacik B, Pamuk ON, Onat AM, Erer SB, Hatemi G, Ozguler Y, et al. Characteristics predicting tuberculosis risk under tumor necrosis factor-α inhibitors: Report from a large Multicenter cohort with high background prevalence. The Journal of Rheumatology. 2016;**43**(3):524-529

[13] Sartori NS, De Andrade NPB, Da Silva Chakr RM. Incidence of tuberculosis in patients receiving anti-TNF therapy for rheumatic diseases: A systematic review. Clinical Rheumatology. 2020;**39**(5):1439-1447

[14] Zhang Z, Fan W, Yang G, Xu Z, Wang J, Cheng Q, et al. Risk of

tuberculosis in patients treated with TNF-α antagonists: A systematic review and meta-analysis of randomised controlled trials. BMJ Open. 2017;**7**(3):e012567

[15] Baddley JW, Cantini F, Goletti D, Gómez-Reino JJ, Mylonakis E, San-Juan R, et al. ESCMID study Group for Infections in compromised hosts (ESGICH) consensus document on the safety of targeted and biological therapies: An infectious diseases perspective (soluble immune effector molecules [I]: Anti-tumor necrosis factor-α agents). Clinical Microbiology and Infection. 2018;**24**:S10-S20

[16] Ozsoy Z, Ozdemir A, Ekici M, Bilgin E, Eken A, Saribas Z, et al. QuantiFERON-TB gold plus for screening and monitoring latent tuberculosis infection in spondyloarthritis patients. Journal of Infection in Developing Countries. 2025;**19**(05):739-746

[17] World Health Organization. Latent Tuberculosis Infection: Updated and Consolidated Guidelines for Programmatic Management [Internet]. Geneva: World Health Organization; 2018. Available from: https://iris.who.int/handle/10665/260233 [Accessed: June 28, 2025]

[18] Wu WT, Chiang MC, Huang YC. The risk of malignancy in patients with psoriasis treated with long-term tumour necrosis factor-alpha inhibitors: A systematic review and meta-analysis. Clinical and Experimental Dermatology. 2025;**50**(5):968-980

[19] Dommasch ED, Abuabara K, Shin DB, Nguyen J, Troxel AB, Gelfand JM. The risk of infection and malignancy with tumor necrosis factor antagonists in adults with psoriatic disease: A systematic review and meta-analysis of randomized controlled trials. Journal of the American Academy of Dermatology. 2011;**64**(6):1035-1050

[20] Xie W, Sun Y, Zhang W, Zhu N, Xiao S. Risk of inflammatory central nervous system diseases after tumor necrosis factor–inhibitor treatment for autoimmune diseases: A systematic review and meta-analysis. JAMA Neurology. 2024;**81**(12):1284

[21] Polachek A, Touma Z, Anderson M, Eder L. Risk of cardiovascular morbidity in patients with psoriatic arthritis: A meta-analysis of observational studies. Arthritis Care and Research. 2017;**69**(1):67-74

[22] Raaby L, Ahlehoff O, De Thurah A. Psoriasis and cardiovascular events: Updating the evidence. Archives of Dermatological Research. 2017;**309**(3):225-228

[23] Yang Z, sheng, Lin N ning, Li L, Li Y. The effect of TNF inhibitors on cardiovascular events in psoriasis and psoriatic arthritis: An updated meta-analysis. Clinical Reviews in Allergy and Immunology. 2016;**51**(2):240-247

[24] Champs B, Degboé Y, Barnetche T, Cantagrel A, Ruyssen-Witrand A, Constantin A. Short-term risk of major adverse cardiovascular events or congestive heart failure in patients with psoriatic arthritis or psoriasis initiating a biological therapy: A meta–analysis of randomised controlled trials. RMD Open. 2019;**5**(1):e000763

[25] Mattay SS, Zamani M, Saturno D, Loftus EV, Ciorba MA, Yarur A, et al. Risk of major adverse cardiovascular events in immune-mediated inflammatory disorders on biologics and small molecules: Network meta-analysis. Clinical Gastroenterology and Hepatology. 2024;**22**(5):961-970.e12

[26] Sun X, Cui Z, Wang Q, Liu L, Ding X, Wang J, et al. Formation and clinical effects of anti-drug antibodies against biologics in psoriasis treatment: An analysis of current evidence. Autoimmunity Reviews. 2024;**23**(4):103530

[27] Bendtzen K, Furst D, Romain P. Tumor Necrosis Factor-Alpha Inhibitors: Induction of Antibodies, Autoantibodies, and Autoimmune Diseases. Wolters Kluwer; 2019

[28] D'Gama JD, Bermas BL. Safety of biologic agents for the management of rheumatic diseases during pregnancy. Current Opinion in Rheumatology. 2024;**36**(3):184-190

[29] Russell MD, Dey M, Flint J, Davie P, Allen A, Crossley A, et al. British Society for Rheumatology guideline on prescribing drugs in pregnancy and breastfeeding: Immunomodulatory anti-rheumatic drugs and corticosteroids. Rheumatology. 2023;**62**(4):e48-e88

[30] Ţiburcă L, Bembea M, Zaha DC, Jurca AD, Vesa CM, Raţiu IA, et al. The treatment with interleukin 17 inhibitors and immune-mediated inflammatory diseases. Current Issues in Molecular Biology. 2022;**44**(5):1851-1866

[31] Shi W, Zhao Z, Zhai Y, Ye X, Xu F. Adverse events associated with IL-23 and IL-12/23 inhibitors in the clinical management of psoriasis: A comprehensive pharmacovigilance analysis. BMC Pharmacology and Toxicology. 2025;**26**(1):11

[32] Davidson L, Van Den Reek JMPA, Bruno M, Van Hunsel F, Herings RMC, Matzaraki V, et al. Risk of candidiasis associated with interleukin-17 inhibitors: A real-world observational study of multiple independent sources. The Lancet Regional Health. Europe. 2022;**13**:100266

[33] Wu KK, Lee MP, Lee EB, Wu JJ. Risk of herpes zoster with IL-17 inhibitor therapy for psoriasis and other inflammatory conditions. Journal of Dermatological Treatment. 2020;**31**(4):359-365

[34] Vassilopoulos A, Thomas K, Vassilopoulos D. Infections in psoriatic arthritis: Association with treatment. Therapeutic Advances in Musculoskeletal Disease. 2024;**16**:1759720X241289201

[35] Androutsakos T, Dimitriadis K, Koutsompina ML, Vassilakis KD, Pouliakis A, Fragoulis GE. Hepatitis B reactivation in PsA patients: An SLR and meta-analysis for IL-17, IL-23 and JAK inhibitors. Rheumatology. 2025;**64**(3):935-942

[36] Li J, Xiang X, Wang Z, Miao C, Chen Y, Xu Z. Safety of interleukin inhibitors in psoriatic patients with latent tuberculosis infection without chemoprophylaxis: A systematic review. Acta Dermato-Venereologica. 2025;**105**:adv42081

[37] Wu S, Xu Y, Yang L, Guo L, Jiang X. Short-term risk and long-term incidence rate of infection and malignancy with IL-17 and IL-23 inhibitors in adult patients with psoriasis and psoriatic arthritis: A systematic review and meta-analysis. Frontiers in Immunology. 2023;**14**:1294416

[38] Krzysztofik M, Brzewski P, Kulbat A, Masajada M, Richter K, Wysocki WM. The IL-23/Th17 pathway inhibitors in the treatment of psoriasis and the risk of skin malignancies: A review. Advances in Dermatology and Allergology. 2024;**41**(6):552-559

[39] Vangilbergen M, Stockman A, Van De Velde A, Garmyn M, Punie K,

Hillary T. The role of interleukin-17 and interleukin-23 inhibitors in the development, progression, and recurrence of cancer: A systematic review. JAAD International. 2024;**17**:71-79

[40] Pina, Vegas L, Le Corvoisier P, Penso L, Paul M, Sbidian E, Claudepierre P. Risk of major adverse cardiovascular events in patients initiating biologics/apremilast for psoriatic arthritis: A nationwide cohort study. Rheumatology. 2022;**61**(4):1589-1599

[41] Shawky AM, Almalki FA, Abdalla AN, Abdelazeem AH, Gouda AM. A comprehensive overview of globally approved JAK inhibitors. Pharmaceutics. 2022;**14**(5):1001

[42] Li X, Hu Q, Xu T. Janus kinase inhibitors and the risk of infections: A network meta-analysis across disease indications. Expert Opinion on Drug Safety. 2025:1-13

[43] Adas MA, Alveyn E, Cook E, Dey M, Galloway JB, Bechman K. The infection risks of JAK inhibition. Expert Review of Clinical Immunology. 2022;**18**(3):253-261

[44] Yang F, Lu C, Wang Y, Liu H, Leng X, Zeng X. Efficacy and safety of Janus kinase inhibitors in patients with psoriasis and psoriatic arthritis: A systematic review and meta-analysis. Clinical Rheumatology. 2023;**42**(6):1593-1605

[45] Xu Q, He L, Yin Y. Risk of herpes zoster associated with JAK inhibitors in immune-mediated inflammatory diseases: A systematic review and network meta-analysis. Frontiers in Pharmacology. 2023;**14**:1241954

[46] Kuo MH, Ko PH, Wang ST, Tseng CW. Incidence of HBV reactivation in psoriasis patients undergoing cytokine inhibitor therapy: A single-Center study and systematic review with a meta-analysis. Viruses. 2024;**17**(1):42

[47] Picchianti-Diamanti A, Aiello A, De Lorenzo C, Migliori GB, Goletti D. Management of tuberculosis risk, screening and preventive therapy in patients with chronic autoimmune arthritis undergoing biotechnological and targeted immunosuppressive agents. Frontiers in Immunology. 2025;**16**:1494283

[48] Evangelatos G, Koulouri V, Iliopoulos A, Fragoulis GE. Tuberculosis and targeted synthetic or biologic DMARDs, beyond tumor necrosis factor inhibitors. Therapeutic Advances in Musculoskeletal Disease. 2020;**12**:1759720X20930116

[49] Russell MD, Stovin C, Alveyn E, Adeyemi O, Chan CKD, Patel V, et al. JAK inhibitors and the risk of malignancy: A meta-analysis across disease indications. Annals of the Rheumatic Diseases. 2023;**82**(8):1059-1067

[50] Stovin C, Russell MD, Alveyn E, Adeyemi O, Patel V, Adas MA, et al. OA08 JAK inhibitors and the risk of malignancy: A meta-analysis across licenced disease indications. Rheumatology. 2023;**62**(Suppl. 2): kead104.008

[51] Elmariah SB, Smith JS, Merola JF. JAK in the [black] box: A dermatology perspective on systemic JAK inhibitor safety. American Journal of Clinical Dermatology. 2022;**23**(4):427-431

[52] Zhao SS, Riley D, Hernandez G, Alam U. Comparative safety of JAK inhibitors versus TNF or IL-17 inhibitors for cardiovascular disease and cancer in psoriatic arthritis and axial spondyloarthritis. Clinical Therapeutics. 2025;**47**(4):293-297

[53] Ytterberg SR, Bhatt DL, Mikuls TR, Koch GG, Fleischmann R, Rivas JL, et al. Cardiovascular and cancer risk with Tofacitinib in rheumatoid arthritis. The New England Journal of Medicine. 2022;**386**(4):316-326

[54] Makris A, Barkas F, Sfikakis PP, Liberopoulos E, Agouridis AP. The effect of Upadacitinib on lipid profile and cardiovascular events: A meta-analysis of randomized controlled trials. Journal of Clinical Medicine. 2022;**11**(23):6894

[55] Rajasimhan S, Pamuk O, Katz JD. Safety of Janus kinase inhibitors in older patients: A focus on the thromboembolic risk. Drugs & Aging. 2020;**37**(8):551-558

[56] Mytheen S, Varghese A, Joy J, Shaji A, Tom AA. Investigating the risk of deep vein thrombosis with JAK inhibitors: A disproportionality analysis using FDA adverse event reporting system database (FAERS). Expert Opinion on Drug Safety. 2023;**22**(10):985-994

[57] Schafer P. Apremilast mechanism of action and application to psoriasis and psoriatic arthritis. Biochemical Pharmacology. 2012;**83**(12):1583-1590

[58] Mavropoulos A, Zafiriou E, Simopoulou T, Brotis AG, Liaskos C, Roussaki-Schulze A, et al. Apremilast increases IL-10-producing regulatory B cells and decreases proinflammatory T cells and innate cells in psoriatic arthritis and psoriasis. Rheumatology. 2019;**58**(12):2240-2250

[59] Chiu HY, Hung YT, Huang YH. Comparative short-term risks of infection and serious infection in patients receiving biologic and small-molecule therapies for psoriasis and psoriatic arthritis: A systemic review and network meta-analysis of randomized controlled trials. Therapeutic Advances in Chronic Disease. 2023;**14**:20406223231206225

[60] Persson R, Cordey M, Paris M, Jick S. Safety of Apremilast in patients with psoriasis and psoriatic arthritis: Findings from the UK clinical practice research datalink. Drug Safety. 2022;**45**(11):1403-1411

[61] Kavanaugh A, Augustin M, Lespessailles E, Papp K, Paris M, Chen R, et al. AB0743 low rates of major adverse cardiac events, malignancies, and serious infections in patients with psoriasis and psoriatic arthritis treated with apremilast for ≥156 weeks: Pooled analysis from the esteem and palace 1-3 phase 3 trials. Annals of the Rheumatic Diseases. 2017;**76**:1314-1315

[62] Kahn JS, Casseres RG, Her MJ, Dumont N, Gottlieb AB, Rosmarin D. Treatment of psoriasis with biologics and Apremilast in patients with a history of malignancy: A retrospective chart review. Journal of Drugs in Dermatology : JDD. 2019;**18**(4):S1545961619P0387X

[63] Persson R, Hagberg KW, Qian Y, Vasilakis-Scaramozza C, Jick S. The risks of major cardiac events among patients with psoriatic arthritis treated with apremilast, biologics, DMARDs or corticosteroids. Rheumatology. 2021;**60**(4):1926-1931

[64] Pina Vegas L, Le Corvoisier P, Penso L, Paul M, Sbidian E, Claudepierre P. POS0201 risk of major adverse cardiovascular events in patients initiating biologics/apremilast for psoriatic arthritis: A Nationwide population-based study using the French health insurance database. Annals of the Rheumatic Diseases. 2021;**80**:317

[65] Hansildaar R, Van Geel EH, Çoban F, Dijkshoorn B, Heslinga M, Bos R, et al. Cardiometabolic effects of Apremilast

in patients with psoriatic arthritis: A prospective cohort study. The Journal of Rheumatology. July 2025;**52**(7):678-686. DOI: 10.3899/jrheum.2024-0791

[66] Ekici M, Apraş BŞ. Psychiatric risk profile of apremilast. Ulusal Romatoloji Dergisi. 2024;**16**(2):87-89

Chapter 6

Psoriasis from Patient's Perspective: Illness Narratives

Columba-Julieta Navarro-Romero, Georgina Vega-Fregoso, Sandra Guzmán-Silahua and Arnulfo-Hernán Nava-Zavala

Abstract

Psoriasis is a chronic, disabling disease not only in terms of physical condition but also psychosocially, which leads to a significant increase in the burden of the disease in all aspects of daily life. This impact goes beyond the patient and affects their circle of interaction, contributing to the deterioration of mental health. The subjective experience of psoriasis has been less studied compared to objective assessments of severity. However, through qualitative research that has been conducted, it has been possible to approach the lived experience of psoriasis from a broader perspective, realistically frame it, and identify the unmet needs of patients and the barriers to accessing adequate and timely care models. Additionally, it allows the recognition of necessary elements for designing more human, fair, and appropriate care strategies. Research from the sociomedical sciences, based on qualitative analysis and contextualized in sociocultural aspects, suggests that the social phenomenon of stigma is a crucial part of what patients endure—this suffering being understood as the experience of psoriasis from the patient's point of view. This stigma stems mainly from a lack of information about the disease among the general population and even within the medical community itself.

Keywords: psoriasis, illness narratives, narrative medicine, qualitative research, sociomedicine

1. Introduction

The way psoriasis has been addressed with the objective of exploration of a subjective approach consists mostly of quantitative approximations aimed at determining metrics associated with quality of life, leaving aside the total experience, suffering, social difficulties, and identity rearrangements to cope with psoriasis. However, these analyses have paved the way for evidencing the need for qualitative research with the objective of gaining a better understanding of patients' unmet needs and thereby improving care strategies.

2. The burden of psoriasis: Exploring the subjective experience

One of the first works intending to explore the subjective world of psoriasis in relation to the clinical characteristics of the disease was carried out in 1997 by Fortune et al. in their study included 150 participants and used clinical severity assessment scales like PASI and quantitative scales on the impacts on the quality of life of people with psoriasis like DLQI, they found that there was no correlation between the severity assessment score and the quality of life impact score. However, the quality of life impact score was higher when the plaque locations were in visible body regions [1].

On the other hand, in the meta-analysis performed with a selection of publications on the clinical severity of the disease and its relationship with psychosocial comorbidity, Kimball et al. found that this psychosocial impact is not always proportional to objective disease severity counts. They concluded that it is essential to include approaches to the psychosocial burden as it plays a primary role in the patient's perception of their severity over the life course [2].

In this decade, the work of Sumpton et al., who conducted a systematic review of publications focused on qualitative analyses of the experiences and perspectives of patients with psoriasis and psoriatic arthritis, found that the disease is an uncontrollable *illness* that determines life decisions and course with significant disruption of social and family roles [3].

The evidence of a subjective *illness experience* of patients with psoriasis is determinant for the course of the disease has led to convening expert group meetings with the objective of sharing information and developing tools to achieve a better approach and understanding of the life journey of patients with psoriasis. These meetings aim to address various elements that interrelate with the *illness* to improve care strategies. From these meetings, the concept of Cumulative Life Course Impairment (CLCI) has been coined, which is presented as a new paradigm for evaluating the impact of psoriasis on patients' quality of life. The goal of CLCI is to achieve a better understanding of the global progressive impact of psoriasis, contributing to identifying patients with greater vulnerability and facilitating the most appropriate and individually tailored treatment decisions. The definition of CLCI is the accumulated result of the balance between the burden of stigmatization, physical and psychological comorbidities, coping strategies, and external factors modulated by the patient's personality style [4]. However, yet, there are no tools or methodologies applicable to the clinical field, accessible to the physician or health personnel, that allow us a systematic evaluation of this CLCI.

In parallel, other qualitative studies have been carried out with other objectives of analysis, such as evaluations of the acceptance of psoriasis in the context of body image, bodily experience, and social support through scales that reveal that acceptance of the disease is positively related to the perception of social support. This demonstrates the lack of relationship between acceptance of the disease and the objective clinical evaluation of severity, highlighting the limitations of the biomedical model and the importance of patients' social context for coping with and accepting their health condition [5].

Research conducted from a qualitative approach has generated knowledge about areas of opportunity for designing strategies for better patient-centered care, as well as pertinent support during the disease.

3. Sociocultural approach to psoriasis

As we have mentioned before, we use the concept of *Illness* instead of the *Disease* concept. What do we mean? In Medical Anthropology, there is a difference between the two.

Illness, according to Arthur Kleinman, refers to the human experience of symptoms and suffering. It refers to how a person experiences illness and how both the person and their family members or social network perceive, live with, and respond to symptoms and disability.

But the personal experience of illness is shaped by collective culture. Our experience of illness and expectations about how to behave when we become ill—and how to respond to someone who is ill—depend on our individual biographies, and on the socially constructed meanings and typification within our environment. Therefore, it differs from person to person [6].

A person with psoriasis gives a particular meaning to their condition, which determines their actions. Healthcare-seeking trajectories are shaped by that meaning and, in most cases, by the metaphors that arise at the moment when the first symptoms appear. For this reason, care is often directed toward a presumed cause that is frequently attributed to infectious, allergic, or even malignant processes such as cancer. Depending on that meaning, the experience of distress and the course of medical attention required by the appearance of visible, scaly, and highly symptomatic skin lesions will vary.

Disease is the health problem from the physician's perspective, based on a biomedical model in which the illness is reconfigured solely as an alteration in biological or functional structure [6].

In specific terms, psoriasis refers to the nosological translation made by the physician based on the interpretation of the clinical aspects of the illness, supported by an interview in which they gather the patient's narratives and integrate them with objective data from physical examination and paraclinical tests. These are mediated by technological tools and incorporated into the physician's theoretical knowledge regarding the disease, it is possible associated risk factors, and their prior experience with psoriasis. This allows the physician to issue a diagnosis and guide treatment actions. However, this is done from a perspective removed from the patient's subjectivity, relying instead on regulatory frameworks such as the evidence-based medicine model.

Finally, *Sickness*, following the concepts developed by Kleinman, refers to the disorder in a generic sense within a population, in relation to macrosocial forces (economic, political, institutional).

Living conditions play a major role in increasing the risk of developing certain illnesses or complications. As previously discussed, psoriasis is associated with a range of comorbidities, such as obesity, metabolic disease, psoriatic arthritis, and mental illness. In biomedical terms, these are linked to a common inflammatory pathophysiological substrate. However, the experience of illness and comorbidities can differ depending on social resources—whether they promote or limit individual development within their social group, their access to care, resource availability for proper management, and lifestyle.

The social experience is embodied in how we feel and live through our bodily states and how we present ourselves to others. It is also shaped by how others respond to these disruptive bodily states, which significantly impacts the lived experience of illness and the actions of the affected person.

The interpretation of symptoms throughout the course of illness is the interpretation of a changing system of meanings that are embodied and can be understood only through interpretation within the context of the person's constructed social references [7].

4. The skin that envelops us

Patients with psoriasis suffer from a visible, symptomatic skin *disease* that afflicts and limits them, but they also suffer from a *disease* whose harmful effects are amplified when interacting with others. Richards et al. reported how divergences in beliefs regarding psoriasis generate greater stress and conflict among the partners of patients with psoriasis, leading them to conclude that it is advisable for couples to be informed jointly about the disease to better understanding and less couple conflicts [8], so it is desirable to include our patients' partners in medical consultation and solve their doubts.

For their part, Utjek et al., in their work on the sociological perspective of the daily life of patients with psoriasis, identify stigma as the distinctive aspect of living with psoriasis, and that people with the *disease* direct coping strategies to contain the stigma, which leads to emotional exhaustion and deteriorates social function [9].

The findings reported by Jankowiak et al., when analyzing the levels of stigmatization of patients with psoriasis according to their clinical and demographic characteristics, found that women feel more stigmatized than men. That is, the phenomenon of stigma and social dysfunction is not a reference to the disease itself, but to the roles in the social group in which one lives. They also report that the presence of psoriasis lesions on the entire skin surface was the only variable that correlated with greater stigmatization [10].

The approaches to the socialization problems of patients with psoriasis that have been carried out by Ghorbanibirgani et al., in whose phenomenological observations account for how rejection and loneliness, lack of social support, feelings of uselessness, together with a weak self-concept, were the emergent themes of the stigma phenomenon. They also observed that coping strategies are aimed at seeking social networks, greater awareness about their *illness* through seeking information, and avoiding the gaze of others. However, experiences are also determined by the beliefs people have about their *illness* or the information available regarding it [11, 12].

5. Psoriasis is felt

The phenomenological analysis conducted by Glynn et al., in women with psoriasis, found that the *illness experience* of patients is significantly determined by subjective symptoms such as itching and burning. These are elements that are rarely considered for assessing the severity of the disease or as a treatment objective. They also report as a relevant finding the patients' concern about therapeutic strategies perceived as good, bad, and dreadful, from which the importance of joint decision-making between physician and patient, centered on the individual needs of each person, is concluded [13].

In relation to the study of subjective symptoms, Ljossa et al., in their work exploring skin pain in psoriasis, found that itching is the most relevant symptom for limiting daily activities, which determines evasive social attitudes and leads to sleep pattern disturbance with detriment to physical health and mental comorbidity such as anxiety and depression [14].

Brogniart L., for his part, in his doctoral work based on grounded theory, found the difficulty of daily life for patients with psoriasis associated with the phenomenon of stigmatization, and that itching is the main symptom affecting the quality of life of patients [15].

6. The skin that reveals emotion

With the objective of understanding the triggering or exacerbating phenomena of the disease, beyond the known risk factors described within the biomedical model, Olivia Hughes, through qualitative research, found that anger is related to sensory perceptions of the skin and that emotions are also closely related to the onset and progression of the disease. That is, negative emotions in people with psoriasis play a primary role as triggers or exacerbators of the disease [16], which was also reported by Guerreiro et al., in Brazil. Their work identifies in the participants' narratives that stress is a trigger for the disease or relapses, physical symptoms such as burning, itching, and joint pain are determinants of limitations in daily life, and the visibility of lesions leads to greater social rejection and isolation as part of the stigma phenomenon [17].

Conversely, Lee Lin et al. found that the physical symptoms of the disease, such as itching and burning, are triggers for the stress experienced by people with psoriasis. They report that patients perceive discrimination and stigmatization and that coping strategies include seeking highly effective treatments, alternative medicine, acceptance of the disease, and coexistence with it in daily life [18].

Regarding some particular clinical variants, Reisner et al. reported that patients with Generalized Pustular Psoriasis identified stress and changes in emotional state as the main trigger. They report that participants perceived that doctors do not recognize or value the physical, mental, and emotional pain of the disease [19].

7. The pain of psoriasis that transcends the skin

Psoriasis, being a disease with different clinical forms and a range of associated comorbidities, implies a burden attributed to skin involvement, but also dependent on the clinical form and associated comorbidities for each patient. With respect to some comorbidities, such as psoriatic arthritis, which is highly prevalent, Erskine et al., in their work based on grounded theory on disease representations, found that beliefs regarding psoriatic arthritis affect the way patients cope with the disease. The emergent themes were: identity (stress, uncertainty), cause (lack of disease control), the disease as a determinant of life decisions, and fear of the consequences of the disease. They also reported that limiting physical symptoms such as pain and lack of joint mobility, mental burden (anxiety, depression), and feelings of shame, in addition to the judgments of others, significantly deteriorate social life. Participants reported how ineffective or inappropriate treatments for daily life generate greater suffering and hopelessness. They also identified a need for joint decision-making with the medical team through patient empowerment [20].

8. The patient's view of psoriasis vs. the doctor's view

Some qualitative studies exploring the different perspectives on psoriasis between patients and primary care physicians, through a comparative phenomenological approach, reported that patients do not trust primary care physicians for the management of their disease due to perceived lack of understanding of their psoriasis disease on the part of the doctors. In contrast, they found that primary doctors assume psoriasis to be a disease with a high physical, emotional, and social impact, but do not consider these to be issues that should be addressed in the consultation. This results in patients perceiving a suboptimal approach to psoriasis severity and inadequate care [21].

Continuing with the exploration of divergences concerning the perception of psoriasis, Bettina Trettin et al., in Denmark, in their phenomenological approach to the follow-up perspective of health professionals and patients, found how patients perceive ambivalence in recommendations. They found that care within the biomedical framework represents a safe reference framework for patients but is incompatible with daily life due to the time, costs, and travel involved. Patients implement strategies to balance treatments, care times, and follow-up in daily life [22].

From another angle and with the objective of exploring the interaction of patients with psoriasis with health personnel, George et al. found that patients experience evasive attitudes from personnel, trivializing the disease and paying little attention to the stigma phenomenon. This represents a great burden for patients because they perceive that they are not offered adequate support by focusing only on the purely clinical elements of the disease [23]. Also, Joy de Vere Hunt et al. evaluated the experience of living with psoriasis in adolescent patients who describe feeling dehumanized by their doctors due to the trivialization of their *illness* related to stigma and social rejection. They also found in their accounts a great concern about the effect of treatments on future life [24]. For their part, Saeedinezhad et al., in Iran, through a phenomenological exploration of the *illness experience* of living with psoriasis, reported that progression to worsening of the disease due to a delay in diagnosis or due to inappropriate or impertinent interventions, due to lack of knowledge of the disease by medical personnel, is a great challenge. The researchers identified disease recurrence as one of the greatest fears and characterized mental and physical *illness* as causing isolation and a greater burden of the disease [25].

9. Illness narratives

During a medical consultation, the patient—through narration—can reframe and contain the chaos caused by illness. Therefore, during the medical-patient interview, the physician can serve as a channel for reflection, reorientation, and action toward improved health, promoting spaces for communication.

The medical encounter takes place in a highly structured setting, where the physician interprets what "the problem" is based on what the patient reports.

Some authors have found that the way in which symptoms and suffering are narrated is important not only for communicating and guiding the search for help, but also because it influences the perception of symptoms and how one copes with illness. It can amplify or lessen the intensity of symptoms and the emotional response to the illness [26].

Narrative reasoning is central to clinical practice because paying attention to patients' stories—their narratives—allows us to access their experiences and life worlds. It helps us understand the patient as an active individual who faces affliction through the meanings that guide their behavior in the face of illness [26]. Therefore, approaching illness through narrative helps to comprehend the patient's experience and understand how their own interpretations shape how they deal with or respond to the illness.

The metaphors used in their stories reflect the cultural context from which they emerge and provide direction for the actions taken to cope with illness and build resilience. Using the knowledge obtained through narratives to guide clinical interventions requires active listening and the creation of spaces that encourage the recounting of stories rooted in the individual's bodily knowledge and lived experience within specific social contexts.

In our work carried out in the Mexican population in western Mexico, from a phenomenological-hermeneutical approach from the perspective of *Illness Narratives*, where *illness* proposes this exploration and recognition of the subjective dimension, the *illness experience* from patients with psoriasis perspective responds to the question of how the individual feels, their experiences, and how it affects their life. This is more than just accounting for the pathological state itself: burning, inflammation, inability to walk, and pain. It is about recognizing those aspects of life with psoriasis that led to the greatest individual, family, and social repercussions for those who suffer from it, and for which support and care strategies can be designed.

The modification of interpersonal relationships due to body alterations affects sexuality, stemming from patients' self-perception as they see their bodies with a dermatological condition that generates shame, feelings of worthlessness, and physical pain, which limits their social interactions to the detriment of couple relationships. The subjective experience of pain also lies in the social limitations that psoriasis imposes on them and the deprivation of their own experiences that are common in the lifeworld of their peers, which contributes to the mental *disease* as depression and anxiety, that is known to be highly prevalent in patients with psoriasis [27].

It has been previously published that, in the United States, absenteeism and low productivity of patients with psoriasis represent an indirect cost of 40% of the total cost of the disease [26]. Our findings suggest that low productivity is influenced not only by disease itself but also by processes associated with medical attention in a social frame of rejection that enhances job instability, which leads to less economic income affecting not only the patient but also the whole family dynamics.

We identify how significantly the disease decisively influences important decisions for future life projects, such as career choice or the limitation of being able to perform expected roles as part of a supportive family or social network, or the management of resources for disease care, which limits the development opportunities for the entire family unit [28].

All the above refers to that three-directional body-mind-spirit relationship where individuals with psoriasis, during their *illness*, suffer bodily, psychic, and social deterioration. This together determines limited, dysfunctional, harmful ways of life and affects their way of being-in-the-world and thereby their intersubjective experience. This suffering or pain leads to a maximum state of not wanting to be in life anymore, which the medical frame defines as suicidality, ranging from ideation-planning-attempt or consummation of suicide. In this way, it is evident that in a feedback loop, the body, mind, and social interaction are crucial in determining emotions and life experience.

People with psoriasis, after the chaos generated by the first symptoms and signs, their daily life restrictions, and their changes in identity roles in Ref. to their self-perceptions, they transcend others in the way others respond and qualify that stigma, that new identity, generating greater suffering or finding supportive social networks that lead to a less harmful experience. Our findings suggest that *Illness* is determined by social interactions, not only by biological disruption itself.

In our research, people with psoriasis perceive a lack of information as a central element of their *illness* experience that permeates all spheres of daily life. Narratives expose, either explicitly or tacitly, that the lack of information causes the phenomenon of stigma, but also the lack of early diagnoses and effective treatments, as well as better job opportunities and alternative ways to care for themselves. This decisively impacts the *illness* experience through the construction of meanings and coping strategies. For example, by believing that it is a contagious *disease*, people are discredited; the affected person assumes themselves as discreditable, devalued, with a *disease* that implies an investment of resources of all kinds. This puts them at a crossroads, such that they seek medical attention either privately or publicly, as this is the socially validated care model for solving health problems [28].

10. Conclusions

Psoriasis is a *disease* that determines a modification of the affected individuals' self-identity. The meanings attributed to psoriasis imply for the social group a physical and moral stigma that makes the individual who suffers from it vulnerable and rejected, marginalized, which generates a greater negative impact on their experience and limits social interaction. The foregoing influences greater mental comorbidity. Furthermore, psoriasis determines that people have fewer opportunities for labor or economic development since, having a physical limitation, they have lower productivity in economic terms, but must also bear the direct or indirect costs of caring for their new health condition.

Qualitative health research offers us an approach to the reality of people within their social environment in which they interact. This allows for the creative and joint design of care strategies and the proposal of public health policies for greater efficiency and relevance of health services.

Acknowledgements

We would like to thank Ximena Ochoa for her collaboration on this publication.

Conflict of interest

The authors declare no conflict of interest.

Author details

Columba-Julieta Navarro-Romero[1,2*], Georgina Vega-Fregoso[2,3], Sandra Guzmán-Silahua[4,5] and Arnulfo-Hernán Nava-Zavala[4,5,6]

1 Department of Dermatology, Mexican Social Security Institute, Guadalajara, Mexico

2 Programa de Maestría en Ciencias Sociomédicas, Department of Sociomedical Sciences, University of Guadalajara, Guadalajara, Mexico

3 Department of Sociomedical Sciences, University of Guadalajara, Guadalajara, Mexico

4 Social, Epidemiologic, and Health Services Research Unit, OOAD State Jalisco, Guadalajara, Mexico

5 International Program, Medicine, Autonomous University of Guadalajara, Guadalajara, Mexico

6 Rheumatology and Immunology Service, Internal Medicine Division, Western General Hospital, Guadalajara, Mexico

*Address all correspondence to: columba_navarro@hotmail.com

References

[1] Fortune DG, Main CJ, O'Sullivan TM, Griffiths CE. Quality of life in patients with psoriasis: The contribution of clinical variables and psoriasis-specific stress. British Journal of Dermatology. 1997;**137**(5):755-760. DOI: 10.1046/j.1365-2133.1997.19472062.x

[2] Kimball AB, Jacobson C, Weiss S, Vreeland MG, Wu Y. The psychosocial burden of psoriasis. American Journal of Clinical Dermatology. 2005;**6**(6): 383-392. DOI: 10.2165/00128071-200506060-00005

[3] Sumpton D, Kelly A, Tunnicliffe DJ, Craig JC, Hassett G, Chessman D, et al. Patients' perspectives and experience of psoriasis and psoriatic arthritis: A systematic review and thematic synthesis of qualitative studies. Arthritis Care and Research. 2020;**72**(5):711-722. DOI: 10.1002/acr.23896

[4] Ros S, Puig L, Carrascosa JM. Discapacidad acumulada en el transcurso vital: La cicatriz de la psoriasis en la vida del paciente. Actas Dermo-Sifiliográficas. 2014;**105**(2):128-134. DOI: 10.1016/j.ad.2013.02.009

[5] Sakson-Obada O, Pawlaczyk M, Gerke K, Adamski Z. Acceptance of psoriasis in the context of body image, body experience, and social support. Health Psychology Report. 2017;**5**(3):251-257. DOI: 10.5114/hpr.2017.63824

[6] Kleinman A. The meaning of symptoms and disorders. In: The Illness Narratives. Suffering, Healing, and the Human Condition. 1st ed. New York: Basic Books, Inc., Publishers; 1998. pp. 3-30

[7] Liz HS. ¿Cómo analizar las narrativas del padecer?: construcción de una propuesta teórico metodológica. Revista CONAMED. 2016;**21**(2):60-65

[8] Richards HL, Fortune DG, Chong SLP, Mason DL, Sweeney SKT, Main CJ, et al. Divergent beliefs about psoriasis are associated with increased psychological distress. Journal of Investigative Dermatology. 2004;**123**(1):49-56. DOI: 10.1111/j.0022-202X.2004.22703.x

[9] Uttjek M, Nygren L, Stenberg B, Dufåker M. Marked by visibility of psoriasis in everyday life. Qualitative Health Research. 2007;**17**(3):364-372. DOI: 10.1177/1049732306297674

[10] Jankowiak B, Krajewska-Kułak E, Jakoniuk M, Khvorik DF. Stigmatization among patients with plaque psoriasis. Journal of Clinical Medicine. 2023;**12**(19):6425. DOI: 10.3390/jcm12196425

[11] Ghorbanibirgani A, Fallahi-Khoshknab M, Zarea K, Abedi H. The lived experience of psoriasis patients from social stigma and rejection: A qualitative study. Iranian Red Crescent Medical Journal. 2016;**18**(7):1-7. DOI: 10.5812/IRCMJ.2789.3

[12] Ghorbanibirgani A, Fallahi-Khoshknab M, Zarea K, Abedi H. The meaning of coping with psoriasis: A phenomenological study. Jundishapur Journal of Chronic Disease Care. 2016;5(4):1-8. DOI: 10.17795/jjcdc-36781

[13] Erin G. Women Living with Psoriasis: A Phenomenological Study. Tesis for Degree of Master in Nursing [Not Published]. Newfoundland: Memorial University of Newfoundland. Library and Archives Canada; 2008

[14] Ljosaa T, Bondevik H, Halvorsen JA, Carr E, Wahl AK. The complex

experience of psoriasis related skin pain: A qualitative study. Scandinavian Journal of Pain. 2020;**20**(3):491-498

[15] Brogniart L. Le vécu des patients atteints de psoriasis: une enquête qualitative en soins primaires. Tesis pour le diplome d'etat de docteur en medicine. France: Faculté de Medicine Henri Warembourg; 2021

[16] Hughes O, Hunter R. Understanding the experiences of anger in the onset and progression of psoriasis: A thematic analysis. Skin Health and Disease. 17 Mar 2022;**2**(4):e111. DOI: 10.1002/ski2.111

[17] Guerreiro T, Rodrigues I, Nogueira L, Távora M. Changes in the daily life of people with psoriasis. A Revista Enfermagem UERJ. 2018;**26**:e28332

[18] Lee LL, Huo AP, Chen SL. Experiences and coping behaviors of patients with psoriasis: A qualitative study. The Journal of Dermatological Treatment. 2023;**34**(1):2193661. DOI: 10.1080/09546634.2023.2193661

[19] Reisner D, Johnsson F, Kotowsky N, Brunette S, Valdecantos W, Eyerich K. Impact of generalized pustular psoriasis from the perspective of people living with the condition: Results of an online survey. American Journal of Clinical Dermatology. 2022;**23**(1):65-71

[20] Erskine G, Dures E, McHugh N, Hewlett S. Exploring the illness representations of people with psoriatic arthritis: A secondary analysis of focus group data. Rheumatology Advances in Practice. 2018;**2**(2):rky023. DOI: 10.1093/rap/rky023

[21] Nelson PA, Barker Z, Griffiths CE, Cordingley L, Chew-Graham CA, IMPACT Team. 'On the surface': A qualitative study of GPs' and patients' perspectives on psoriasis. BMC Family Practice. 2013;**14**:158. DOI: 10.1186/1471-2296-14-158

[22] Trettin B, Feldman S, Andersen F, Danbjorg D, Agerskov H. Improving management of psoriasis patients receiving biological treatment: A qualitative approach. Nursing Open. 2021;**8**:1283-1291. DOI: 10.1002/nop2.745

[23] George C, Sutcliffe S, Scheinmann D, Mizara A, McBride SR. Psoriasis: The skin I'm In. Development of a behavior change tool to improve the care and lives of people with psoriasis. Clinical and Experimental Dermatology. 2021;**46**(5):888-895

[24] IVeera Hunt IJ d, McNiven A, Roberts A, Parmar H, McPherson T. 'Not just a piece of skin in front of you'—A qualitative exploration of the experiences of adolescents with eczema and psoriasis with healthcare professionals. BMJ Open. 2021;**11**(1):e041108. DOI: 10.1136/bmjopen-2020-041108

[25] Saeedinezhad F, Dahmardeh H, Yaghoubinia F, Zamani HZ, J. Exploring the experiences of patients with psoriasis: A phenomenological study. Medical-Surgical Nursing Journal. 2022;**11**(3):e135520. DOI: 10.5812/msnj-135520

[26] Laurence K, Ana G, Ekaterina S, Eduardo G. Narrative Medicine. In: Person Centered Medicine. Switzerland. Chapter 14: Springer; 2023. pp. 235-255

[27] Kimball AB, Bensimon AG, Guerin A, Yu AP, Wu EQ, Okun MM, et al. Efficacy and safety of adalimumab among patients with moderate to severe psoriasis with co-morbidities: Subanalysis of results from a randomized, double-blind, placebo-controlled, phase III trial. American Journal of Clinical Dermatology. 1 Feb 2011;**12**(1):51-62.

DOI: 10.2165/11530640-000000000-00000

[28] Navarro C, Vega G, Nava A. Piel y Experiencia: Narrativas del Padecer en Pacientes Con Psoriasis. Tesis for Degree of Master in Sociomedical Sciences [Not Published]. Guadalajara: Universidad de Guadalajara; 2025